The Complete Guide to Intermittent Fasting

Lose fat, build muscle, get toned using IF, Keto and more.

Peter Jackman

Table of Contents

Introduction – Is Fasting Fact or Fad?

Intermittent fasting seems to be the latest in an inexhaustible list of diets of the moment. In diets' wake, we've had every nuance imaginable, literally from A to Z – Atkins to Zone – yet each with one thing in common. They do not achieve their ultimate goal, which is long term, sustained weight loss.

Yet, fasting is different.

Rather than being the latest fad diet kid on the block, it is, in reality, the world's oldest medical treatment. In fact, the father of medicine, Hippocrates, advocated fasting over medication, once saying . . . *"Instead of medicine, fast for a day."*

Did you know that when they are unwell, animals refrain from eating? They do this in the instinctive knowledge that not eating, has a powerful healing effect on the body. For thousands of years this, too, has been known by humans, but unfortunately forgotten more of late.

Yet, it is only within the last few decades that researchers have been able to produce the science to prove the powerful effect of fasting on human health. As a result, fasting is being recognized as a legitimate breakthrough in the fields of weight loss, lean muscle increase, anti-aging, and overall well-being.

Fasting is, of course, an emotive word. Many people associate it with political protest, religious rites or what you do before some surgical procedures. Few people, before the publicity surrounding Intermittent Fasting (IF), considered it as a viable, let-alone a scientific, way to lose weight.

Similarly, when it comes to building muscle, it would seem that not eating is the last thing you'd want to do. After all, we've been conditioned to believe that we've got to mega-dose on protein to *beef* up. It's hardly surprising, then, that there's a great deal of confusion surrounding the concept of IF for building muscle.

At its core, of course, IF is very simple… Fasting simply means not eating. How hard can that be?

Yet, like most, things, the beauty is in the detail. There are many ways to go about it, each one with different effects and outcomes. Small tweaks can make a huge difference. If you go into it blindly, you can pretty much guarantee that you are not going to get the results you desire. However, this book is designed to provide you with an all-encompassing resource to allow you to implement IF as a seamless, continuous lifestyle habit, suited specifically to your individual needs.

In **Part One**, I'll help you cut through all of the white noise to provide a definitive answer to the question, what exactly is IF? Then we will delve into the scientific evidence to substantiate each area of positive impact that the simple act of fasting can have on your body.

In **Part Two**, you will explore each of the different intermittent fasting variants and clarify what specific goals each one is geared towards so you can choose which one will work best for you. We also get into the weeds to produce definitive answers to the questions that can make or break your fasting efforts.

These include . . .

- What to eat during your feeding windows?
- How can you maximize muscle gain while fasting?
- Should you pair intermittent fasting with the ketogenic diet?
- What is the most effective way to fast for fat loss?

Then, in **Part Three**, you will look at what you need to do to make intermittent fasting work specifically for you. After all, it doesn't matter how effective an eating program is, unless you address and overcome the behaviors, thought patterns and habits that have been previously blocked your success. That's why this section will provide you with the tools you need to implement life-long changes that will lead you achieve success. These tools will prevent you from falling back into old routines and habits and instead allow you to reach your goal, be it long term sustainable weight loss, muscle gain, overall health improvement or a combination of all three.

Part One – Intermittent Fasting 101

Chapter 1 – What is IF?

Intermittent Fasting is an eating plan that revolves around strategically not eating for timed periods, either every day or several times a week. This is done to promote positive adaptations in the body that lead to specific outcomes.

It is not a diet in that it does not stipulate a reduced daily caloric count (though this usually results anyway). Rather, intermittent fasting is a lifestyle pattern that is designed to be followed over the long-term.

Many assert that fasting is an unwise choice because it slows down the metabolism, which will lead to lower caloric burn and inevitable fat gain. However, science has shown that this is simply untrue. While starvation is unhealthy, intermittent fasting is about as far removed from starvation as you can get. You still eat, you just increase the gaps between.

Another misconception concerning fasting is that it results in low glucose levels in the bloodstream, which can put a person into a hypoglycemic state. In this state, the body craves simple carbohydrates to get itself out of its weakened, fatigued state. But, once again, the hard, cold facts of science do not back up this belief.

The reality is that going for up to twenty hours without food will not cause a hypoglycemic response. You will have a lowered blood sugar level. But the body responds to this by releasing glycogen which is stored in your muscle cells, into the bloodstream. Which, as you will find out in later chapters, is positive.

Many people, especially, those who have worked hard to add muscle to their body, are concerned that intermittent fasting will lead to loss of lean muscle tissue. On the face of it, it appears to be a legitimate concern. More muscle requires more energy to sustain it. And energy usually comes primarily from food.

However, fasting has been shown to trigger the release of growth hormone, which is one of the most anabolic (muscle building) compounds in your body. One of the things that growth hormone does is to promote the burning of stored body fat, rather than stored muscle tissue, to provide your body with its energy needs. Therefore those with concerns about IF and muscle toning/building can be reassured that IF will also work for them.

How effective is fasting at boosting growth hormone levels? In one study, people had their growth hormone levels tested before and after a 24-hour fast. At the end of the day, the average growth hormone level had increased by a staggering 1,300 percent in female study participants and 2000 percent in males!

How IF *Really* Works

There are many variants of IF, which we will detail in the next section. Each of them is based on the concept of going for a set length of time without food, then eating during a short *feeding window*. This is then repeated. It is intended as a long-term lifestyle choice rather than a short-term diet.

The body of any living being can be in one of two states:

- Fasted
- Fed

These two states are, obviously, counters to one another. To borrow a Chinese concept, they are the *Ying and Yang* of your body. You need both to balance each other.

Fasting affects the body in three positive key ways:

- It optimizes your body's hormonal response.
- It boosts growth hormone release.
- It allows the body to properly digest and absorb vital nutrients.

Let's consider each of these a little more closely.

Hormonal Response

Your hormones are like the orchestra conductors of your body. Every second they regulate the millions of bodily functions that are taking place. Hormones are simply chemical messengers that tell your body's cells what to do. Every single thing you do, from breathing to storing body fat, is controlled by your hormones. Anything you can do to promote the release of beneficial hormones, whilst at the same time, diminish the release of those that promote fat storage and muscle catabolism (destructive metabolism), is going to be positive for your health.

When you fast, certain hormones are enabled, while others are diminished. Two hormones that are released by the pancreas are particularly affected. These are . . .

- Insulin
- Glucagon

Both of these hormones regulate blood sugar levels but they have opposite functions. Insulin transports nutrients into the cell, whereas, glucagon pulls nutrients out of the cell, including fatty acids to be used as energy. Of course, you want your body to use up fat for energy rather than storing it in different cells. And, you guessed it, when you are in a fasted state Glucagon release is optimized.

On the other hand, insulin is released every time you eat. Every morsel that you put into your mouth releases glucose into the bloodstream. This triggers the release of insulin from the pancreas. Insulin has one job; to transport the glucose from the blood into the muscle cell to provide energy. The process that results creates adenosine triphosphate (ATP). It is a chemical that provides energy to drive many processes in our bodies.

For insulin to get into your cells it has to first pass through an insulin regulator. This is your body's version of a doorman that controls who and who doesn't come into a club. Insulin is a bit like a celebrity. It gets the red-carpet treatment and gets to go straight in.

For many people, however, it doesn't work that way. That's because they have become insulin resistant. There is already so much glucose flushed through their cells that the insulin receptors refuse to let any more in. The club is already at full capacity!

However, it gets even worse. Over time your cells automatically become insulin resistant. That means that, even when your cells are low on glycogen, the cells STILL won't accept the insulin, along with the glucose that it is transporting.

The glucose that gets kicked back from the cells is returned to the blood. How does the body react to this? Naturally, it causes the pancreas to release more insulin. This then leads to an excess of, not just glucose, but also insulin, coursing through your system.

Where does the excess glucose go?

It gets stored as body fat around your bodily organs. This is a particularly dangerous type of adipose tissue known as visceral body fat.

Yet, what was it that caused all of this to start in the first place?

Eating – usually too much, too often.

When you don't eat, you do not stimulate the release of insulin. Instead, you encourage the pancreas to release its opposite – glucagon. Which in turn helps to keep the balance.

<u>Growth Hormone Release</u>
Growth hormone, also known as somatotropin, is a protein hormone that is made up of 191 amino acids. It is released by somatropin cells located in the anterior pituitary gland. The growth hormone is an important component of human development, making it vital for the muscle-building process. It is also an important fat-burning hormone.

Just check out what optimized levels of growth hormone can do for your body:

- Increased muscle strength.
- Enhanced fracture healing.
- Boosted weight loss.
- Increased bone strength.
- Lowered risk of cardiovascular disease.
- Enhanced virility.
- Improved cognitive functioning.
- Better sleep.

However, when you have high levels of glucose in your blood, the pancreas not only releases insulin, it also releases a chemical called somatostatin. It has the opposite effect on human growth hormone, and besides, suppresses its production. As a result, the more times that you eat through your day, the less growth hormone you will release into your body. The opposite is also true – the fewer times you eat, the more growth hormone your body will produce.

Digestion & Nutrient Absorption

No matter how hard we try, it is virtually impossible to avoid putting toxins into our bodies. They are contained in the foods that we eat and in the air that we breathe. One effect of toxin overload is that our intestines become clogged up. This limits our ability to efficiently absorb the beneficial nutrients in the food that we eat. When we account for the fact that the majority of health-promoting vitamins and minerals in our foods have already been removed through processing, this is a major concern. It means that we are only getting a fraction of the goodness out of our foods that our bodies deserve.

Many people also fail to properly digest the food that they eat. This can be a result of many factors including not sufficiently hydrating; eating too quickly; not chewing food sufficiently; not eating the sorts of foods that stimulate digestive enzymes; over-indulging in processed foods that the body cannot digest or remove from the body.

All of this results in a build-up of undigested and nutrient bare food in our digestive system. Our body will react to this by creating a build-up of mucus, which weighs us down, makes us feel sluggish and further complicates the digestive process.

In his book, **Colon Health: the Key to a Vibrant Life**, Norman W. Walker, Ph.D. states, *"the elimination of undigested food and other waste products is equally as important as the proper digestion and assimilation of food. Infirmity and sickness, at any age, is the direct result of loading up the body with food, which contains no vitality, and at the same time allowing the intestine to remain loaded with waste matter."*

When you give your body an extended period in which it does not have to digest food, it's a little like shutting down your kitchen to give it a thorough deep clean. And just as you apply cleaners and disinfectants to the oven and dishwasher, so your body releases its own natural cleaners. These are known as macrophages, cells that attack toxins, along with white blood cells that also destroy toxins.

It is only when you are in a fasted state that you can efficiently get rid of the toxins and waste matter that are clogging up your body.

Chapter 2 – Huge Benefits of Intermittent Fasting

Fat Burning

By far the number one reason that people begin to follow the intermittent fasting lifestyle is to lose body fat. The reason that IF (the trending term you will hear for Intermittent Fasting) has become so popular as a weight-loss method is down to three things;

- It works.
- It has scientific backing.
- It requires no expensive food deliveries or subscriptions to dieting clubs.

Your body has two energy systems that it can call upon.

The primary energy system is glucose-based. It relies on carbohydrates to provide this glucose which gets transported in the muscle cell to be converted into adenosine triphosphate. When you consume too many simple carbohydrates, the excess is stored as reserve energy in the form of body fat.

When your body's glucose stores are used up, it turns to its secondary energy system. This is stored body fat, which is a more efficient form of energy than glucose. A byproduct of the fat burning for energy process is a compound known as ketones.

Once you eat a meal, it takes between eight and twelve hours to use up glycogen stores released from that food.

Only then will your body be able to tap into its reserve energy system – stored body fat. Of course, most people's everyday eating pattern never allows them to go for a whole twelve hours without eating. As a result, you never really get to deplete your body's glycogen levels to the point where fat burning kicks in.

Yet, when you do allow your body enough time to expend the body's glycogen stores, it will have no choice but to switch to its secondary energy system. In the process, you will lose the craving to eat sugary simple carbohydrates – a definite plus! This is because your body will be depending on stored body fat and not carbohydrates for the energy that you need to function. Fat is a slow-burning fuel that provides you with a sustained and controlled energy source. Every gram of fat contains 9 calories, compared with just 4 calories per gram of carbohydrate.

An interesting study, published in the journal, *Cell Metabolism*, showed the power of IF as a catalyst for fat loss. The study looked at the effect of different eating protocols on the health of mice. One group of mice could eat whenever they wanted, while the other group was restricted to a specific eating window. At the end of the 38-week trial, the group who were allowed free reign to eat whenever they wanted had become obese and displayed metabolic dysfunction. The group that was restricted to a specific eating window remained normal weight and healthy.

Interestingly both groups ate the same foods and consumed the same total caloric amount each day!

But that wasn't the end of this study. When the mice who were given an eating window were allowed to eat whatever they wanted and to the extent that they desired, they still

DID NOT gain weight. Then when they were allowed to eat at any time of the day on what the scientists deemed their *weekends*, they still managed to maintain their same weight. What this shows is that a person doing IF can have a *cheat day* on the weekend and still not negatively impact their weight loss goals.

The study also looked at the ability of IF to help people who are already obese. It was found that the practice of restricting your caloric intake to a specific time window each day was able to reverse many of the harmful markers associated with obesity. Markers for diabetes, LDL cholesterol, and fatty liver all came down significantly.

So, just how effective is intermittent fasting when it comes to burning body fat? A study from 2014 revealed that IF was able to cause a water loss of between 3-8 percent over 3-24 weeks. During that same time, there was a reduction in waist circumference of 4-7 percent. This indicates that there was a significant loss in dangerous abdominal body fat. This is what is known as visceral body fat. It is the most dangerous form of fat because it surrounds vital bodily organs.

IF also results in fewer overall calories being consumed over the day. It will have you skipping at least one full meal per day, usually, breakfast. Very few people will eat enough calories during their eating window to compensate for the lowered caloric intake. You don't even have to count calories, which is usually an unsustainable long-term strategy, to cut your daily caloric count. Simply skipping a meal is far easier – and it is something that you can quite easily do for the rest of your life!

Another great benefit of IF, as a means of fat loss, is that it allows you to lose body fat without losing muscle tissue.

Traditional dieting is notorious for the collateral muscle tissue that gets lost as you cut back on calories. A study that was reported in the journal, *Obesity Reviews,* revealed that using IF results in significantly reduced levels of muscle loss than traditional forms of dieting. It was shown that traditional dieting by caloric restriction results in 75 percent fat loss and 25 percent muscle tissue loss. With intermittent fasting, those percentages change significantly – 90 percent from body fat and just 10 percent from muscle tissue.

It is important to keep in mind that these results were relevant to people who were not doing any exercise. Resistance training preserves muscle tissue. So, if you are adopting an intermittent fasting lifestyle and doing regular weight training you will be able to maximize fat loss without losing any muscle at all!

Intermittent fasting also boosts your metabolic rate. This means that you will burn more calories even while at rest. We have already mentioned the impact that fasting has on your insulin and glucagon levels. However, it also increases the levels of norepinephrine. This hormone gets sent by the central nervous system to your fat cells and has the effect of stimulating the breakdown of fatty acids to make the production of energy from stored body fat more efficiently.

The evidence makes it abundantly clear that IF is the most efficient, sustainable and easy to adopt a method of fat loss that exists.

Growth Hormone Production

We have already highlighted the fact that IF naturally increases the release of human growth hormone (HGH) by the pituitary gland. Let's now dig a little deeper into this subject.

HGH is released by the pituitary gland in bursts and then directed into the bloodstream. The body will release more HGH after exercise, while you sleep and following a traumatic event.

HGH is transversely related to insulin. Insulin is produced by the pancreas. It has the job of transporting insulin to your muscle cells. When insulin is released into the bloodstream, the body will not release HGH. It is only when insulin has been cleared out that HGH can be secreted. The times when you are assured to have no insulin in your bloodstream are when you are well into a fast and when you are sleeping.

Research has shown that the ideal condition for maximized HGH release in adults is to be in a fasted state. In a study conducted by the American College of Cardiology, fasting resulted in a 1,300 percent increase in HGH release in women and a 2,000 percent increase in men.

The results of that study are astounding. When you consider that hundreds of thousands of men, in particular, are risking their health to take synthetic versions of HGH to boost their muscle-building potential. It makes you wonder why more guys, and women for that fact, aren't following an intermittent fasting lifestyle to build muscle. The answer in many cases is because they don't know about it. They may have heard that IF is an effective way to lose fat but still operate on the mistaken impression that it will cause them to lose muscle tissue.

While we are on the subject of muscle gain, there is another, potentially even more powerful reason to adopt an IF lifestyle. Your body contains a protein called the mammalian target of rapamycin (mTOR). It has been recently revealed to regulate the construction and rejuvenation of muscle tissue.

The activation of mTOR leads to muscle growth because of its ability to enhance protein synthesis. However, if you have too much mTOR coursing through your system, it can have the opposite effect. mTOR is activated by the release of insulin and intense exercise. When you start to work out, mTOR is suppressed. It's only when you have a post-workout meal that it is released.

The really interesting thing is that the way to maximize mTOR release is to firstly suppress it. An extremely effective way to do this is to go on a fast. Combining fasting with exercise is the gold standard when it comes to boosting mTOR release.

Because insulin also causes the release of mTOR, elevated levels of insulin caused by frequent eating of simple carbohydrates can lead to both insulin and mTOR resistance. This is why people with elevated levels of insulin will find it extremely difficult to build muscle.

The best way to bring down your insulin levels is to fast.

Brain Function

The human brain is the only living organ that strives to understand itself. Our understanding of the human brain has undergone some profound changes in recent times. It used to be thought that the brain was static and unable to be changed. Now we know differently.

The brain can constantly adapt and change. The term neuroplasticity has been coined to describe the ability of the brain to form new connections. The brain can also heal itself. New brain connections are facilitated by a family of proteins known as neurotrophic factors. One specific neurotrophic factor has been identified as the most crucial. It is called brain-derived neurotrophic factor (BDNF).

BDNF activates brain stem cells to produce new brain cells. So, the more BDNF you have, the greater your potential to increase the number of brain cells. So, what can you do to maximize your body's production of BDNF? – Intermittent Fasting!

And IF does not increase BDNF just by a little bit! IF has been shown to increase BDNF production by between 50 and 400 percent!

BDNF is most effective at boosting brain cell capacity in the area of the brain called the hippocampus. This area is responsible for long term memory and spatial navigation. As a result, taking on an IF lifestyle is one of the best things you can do to boost your memory, enhance learning capability and control your mood.

Yet, there's more…

The more BDNF you have coursing through your body, the lower your likelihood to suffer from Alzheimer's or Parkinson's diseases. This special protein can protect brain cells from degenerative disorders.

The National Institute of Aging conducted a study on mice that were put on an IF plan. Mark Mattson was a senior investigator on the study and reported that, *"Fasting begun in middle age delayed the onset of memory problems by about six months. This is a large effect, perhaps equivalent to about twenty years in humans."*

In another study, mice that were put on an IF plan began to develop signs of Alzheimer's at the age of two. In human terms, that is around ninety years of age. Mice will normally start showing signs of dementia at 12 months of age, or the equivalent of 45 in human terms.

What this information reveals is that adopting an intermittent fasting lifestyle has the potential to delay the onset of Alzheimer's and other dementia-related conditions by more than four decades!

Interestingly, when the mice were put on a junk food diet with no time restrictions, they began to develop signs of dementia after just nine months. That is yet another powerful reason to adopt healthier eating combined with an IF lifestyle.

The brain-boosting benefits of IF are both impressive and powerful long-term motivators. Especially motivating is that IF results in increased levels of BDNF, meaning we can work to avoid dementia-related illnesses in later life!

As we've already discovered, fasting allows your body to switch from a glucose-based energy system to a fat-based energy system. There is a lot of research attesting to the fact that the brain operates far more efficiently on a fat-based energy system. Most of this research conducted put subjects on the ketogenic diet, which also allows the body to switch to a fat-based energy system.

A 2010 study, which was published in the journal, *Neurobiological Aging*, had 23 people with mild cognitive impairment divided into two groups. The first group followed a ketogenic diet with between 5 and 10 percent of calories coming from carbohydrates. The second group consumed 50 percent of their daily calories from carb sources. The study was carried out over six weeks.

At the end of the study period, the verbal memory skills of those who were operating off a fat-burning energy system (the ketogenic group) were higher than the glucose-based group. Also, the memory recall of the fat-based energy group was significantly better than the other.

A 2005 study focused on the effects of a fat-based energy system on Parkinson's disease. Five people with Parkinson's were put on a ketogenic diet for twenty-eight days. Their Unified Parkinson's Disease Rating Scale (UPDRS) was taken at the beginning of the study and again at weekly intervals. The five subjects who completed the study reduced their UPDRS scores by an average of 10.72 points, which represented an average decrease of nearly 45 percent (a range from 21 to 81 percent) in just twenty-eight days. Resting tremors, balance, gait, mood, and energy level all improved.

A fat-based energy system has also been seen to be ideal for people who are suffering from traumatic brain injury (TBI). People who suffer from TBI are unable to efficiently metabolize glucose for several months after their injury. However, they can make full use of fat for energy. Not only that, but the enhanced production of BDNF also speeds up the brain repair process.

Increased Lifespan and Longevity

There is a lot of research going on regarding slowing down the aging process. The shining star of all of this research is undoubtedly IF. One of the most interesting facts to emerge from this research was that the body reacts to fasting the same way that it does to exercise. Both of them place stress on the body. But the stresses that come from fasting and exercise are considered positive stressors.

When cells are put under mild positive stress, they respond by adapting to cope with the stress. This increased resistance to stress allows the body to better cope with the aging process.

According to Mark Mattson of the National Institute of Aging, *"Intermittent fasting increases lifespan and protects various tissues against disease, in part by Hormesis mechanisms that increase cellular stress resistance. A primary reason that intermittent fasting promotes longevity has to do with the switch to a fat-burning energy system. Fat is a far cleaner form of energy than glucose. As a result, it improves insulin sensitivity. There is a lot less free radical stress than when your body is burning glucose for energy. That means a huge reduction in cellular damage."*

Our bodily organs operate more efficiently when they receive their energy from fat as opposed to glucose. So, as we've already discovered, does the brain. When you are in the fat-burning state of ketosis, the liver produces a compound called beta-hydroxybutyrate (BHB). This is an efficient source of fuel for the brain. BHB is also great for the immune system. It results in a reduced inflammatory response. What's more, research out of the Yale School of Medicine, showed BHB has the effect of recycling damaged immune cells and regenerating new healthy immune cells.

Intermittent fasting was shown to improve many age-related factors, shown in a study that was published in the journal, *Cell Metabolism*. These include rejuvenating the immune system and reducing the cancer risk. It also promotes neurogenesis of the hippocampus and boosts overall cognitive enhancement.

Studies on both mice and humans have shown that intermittent fasting improves longevity by:

- Reducing visceral body fat.
- Lowering the incidence of inflammatory disease.
- Enhancing brain function.
- Increasing bone density.
- Improving memory.

And, best of all, these benefits come without any of the usual side effects that can be associated with prescribed medications.

Chapter 3 – How IF Achieves Incredible Results

<u>The Stone Cold Facts</u>
A study that was published in the journal, *Cell Stem Cell*, revealed that IF activated particular pathways in the body that enables cells to become stronger and more able to resist toxins. This was seen to reduce immune system weakness and help to alleviate age-related diseases.

Intermittent fasting has also been shown to increase the regeneration of stem cells. It activates stem cells to promote self-renewal. In other words, they can divide and make more stem cells. As a result, the body can regenerate.

One factor which leads to stem cell regeneration is that IF reduces the amount of IGF-1 (Insulin-like growth factor 1). This hormone acts similarly to insulin. Lowered insulin and IGF-1 levels promote stem cell regeneration. At the same time, there is immunosuppression of cancer cells.

IF has also been shown to bring about positive changes to the gut biome. Your digestive system consists of some 100 trillion cells. Bacteria outnumber other cells by a ratio of 10:1. Your gut biome is constantly changing following your dietary and lifestyle choices. The healthier your choices, the greater the ratio of good versus bad bacteria.

Not surprisingly, your eating habits have the greatest impact on your gut biome. Intermittent fasting is one of the best things you can do to positively alter your gut bacteria balance. Your gut microflora makes up 80 percent of your immune system. As a result, the positive changes to your gut bacteria will have a profound effect on your immune system. A healthier gut biome will also allow you to sleep more soundly, have greater energy and better concentration.

Improved Hormone & Chemical Sensitivity

Insulin

Insulin is a transportation hormone that carries glucose from the bloodstream to our cells, the glucose is then used to provide energy. When you consume more sugar than your body needs, insulin transports it to your liver for storage. When this storage facility is filled, the excess is stored as body fat.

Insulin is a fat-storage hormone. Not only does it tell fat to store itself in your body, but it also prevents stored fat from being broken down for energy. Too much insulin in the body, then, is bad news if you want to minimize your fat storage.

Every time you eat food, your body will release insulin. This provides it with a ready source of new energy. As a result, it will have absolutely no desire or inclination to use up any of its stored energy. When people are eating carb-laden foods all day long, they will be constantly releasing insulin.

After a prolonged period, your body will stop responding to insulin. The levels of sugar in the blood will not go down. This will cause the pancreas to release even more insulin. A vicious cycle is set up with more insulin leading to greater insulin resistance. This leads to a condition called hyperinsulinemia, characterized by a dangerously high level of blood sugar. Not only is a person with this condition extremely unhealthy, but they are also not able to burn body fat. That is because they have a constant surplus of energy.

The startling truth is that 40 percent of the American population are insulin resistant. That equates to around 130 million people.

So, how do you reduce your levels of insulin? – You do so by not eating!

The only time your body can begin to burn it's body fat stores is when you're not eating. That is when your body can make use of the reserves of energy that are lying around in your body. A study that was published in the *International Journal of Obesity* said intermittent fasting was seen to reduce inflammation, improve metabolic disease markers and reduce insulin resistance.

When you provide a break from eating for your body, you allow it to normalize its blood sugar levels. When we don't have sugar constantly flowing into the bloodstream, we won't be releasing new insulin. We will also be providing the body with the opportunity to draw upon its stored energy in the form of body fat for the energy that we need to function.

One of the most important things you can do to overcome insulin resistance is to follow an IF lifestyle. Inflammation and high triglyceride levels are contributing factors to insulin resistance. These conditions are alleviated when you follow an IF lifestyle.

Leptin

Leptin is another hormone that is positively impacted by IF. It is sometimes called the satiety hormone as it tells us when to be full of food. Every time you eat, leptin is released by the fat cells. It gets transported to the hypothalamus in the brain, which sends the signal that your body is full and no longer needs to eat.

Without leptin, we'd be constantly craving food. Conversely, higher levels of leptin will decrease your feelings of hunger while also speeding up your metabolism. In a healthy person, leptin levels are on the lower level. Food is rewarding when you eat, and after your meal, your leptin levels are increased to signal fullness. There is some data from studies showing that IF can increase leptin production, therefore making you feel fuller faster when eating. The result being weight loss – due to the consumption of less food and fewer calories.

The reduced weight that comes with intermittent fasting will also help to regulate leptin levels.

Normalized Ghrelin Levels

Ghrelin is the *ying* to leptin's *yang*. It is the hormone that tells your brain that you are hungry. In normal situations, our ghrelin levels are high before we eat and low after we have eaten.

The less frequently we eat, the higher the levels of ghrelin we will produce and when you start fasting this can be difficult as you constantly feel hungry. However, your ghrelin levels will usually peak at day 1-2 of fasting, and then after, steadily begin to decline with feelings of pangs of hunger less prominent after day 2.

Another interesting benefit to IF is the higher your ghrelin levels, the higher your levels of growth hormone. Growth hormone promotes muscle growth and increases fat burn. Working out when your ghrelin levels are elevated will boost your growth hormone levels even further.

It has also been shown that high levels of ghrelin in the body will make us better learners. The bottom line here is that high levels of ghrelin release are good for us in a whole raft of ways. And the best way to promote the release of ghrelin is to follow an IF lifestyle.

The old myth that breakfast is the most important meal of the day is undermined by the fact that eating in the early morning is one of the most effective ways to suppress ghrelin. By simply postponing your first meal of the day until around 11 am, you will be able to optimize your ghrelin (and therefore your growth hormone) release.

Inflammation

Inflammation is a natural bodily response to toxins and tissue damage. Acute inflammation is normal and healthy. It is responsible for sending out white blood cells and other chemicals to fight off invaders and help in the healing process. But chronic inflammation is something else entirely.

Chronic inflammation causes damage to your bodily tissues and can result in potentially life-threatening diseases. It is the precursor to almost every disease you can imagine.

So, what causes chronic inflammation?

It is primarily a lifestyle condition. Consuming too much sugar, having an omega fatty acid intake that is heavily weighted toward omega-6 as opposed to omega-3, not exercising and having too much stress in your life are all contributing factors.

IF and exercise is the best way to reduce chronic inflammation. Both of these things improve the levels of Brain-Derived Neurotrophic Factor (BDNF), which is low in people who have chronic inflammation. Enhanced BDNF levels enhance cognitive functioning. It allows old nerve cells to form dense, interconnected webs that significantly improve brain functionality.

BDNF can only be elevated in the brain when inflammation is low. So, the higher the levels of BDNF the lower the level of chronic inflammation.

A study that was published in the journal, *Nutritional Research*, investigated the effect that fasting had on Muslim men during the holy month of Ramadan. During this time, people fast for around twelve hours each day. The conclusion to the study stated, *"These results indicate that RIF [Ramadan Induced Fasting] attenuates inflammatory status of the body by suppressing pro-inflammatory cytokine expression and decreasing body fat and circulating levels of leukocytes."*

Heart Health

When it comes to measuring the health of your heart, medical experts focus on the following factors:

- Cholesterol levels
- Triglyceride levels
- Blood pressure

- Inflammatory markers

It is now a fact that intermittent fasting significantly improves each of these heart health markers. One study, published in the *Journal of Nutritional Biochemistry*, specifically focused on the effects of fasting on the cardiovascular system. Lead researcher, Mark Mattson, concluded the following, *"Enhance cardiovascular and brain functions and improve several risk factors for coronary artery disease and stroke including a reduction in blood pressure and increased insulin sensitivity. Cardiovascular stress adaptation is improved and heart rate variability is increased."*

The study revealed that IF has a great ability to protect the heart and the brain from what is known as ischemic injury. This is a restriction in the blood supply to the tissues of the body. This results in a shortage of glucose and oxygen for the vital cellular metabolic processes that keep the tissues alive.

The transportation of oxygen throughout the body happens through the blood. Restriction of blood supply then leads to a depletion of oxygen supply to the organs of the body. The heart, however, requires a constant supply of oxygen. If blood flow to the heart is restricted for as little as three minutes, a person can suffer from irreversible damage. The same is true of the brain.

A major contributor to the reduced blood supply to the heart is the condition called atherosclerosis. This condition is typified by a build-up of cholesterol and plaque in the arteries which causes blockages that restrict the blood supply. This, in turn, leads to ischemic heart disease.

Finding a way to enhance blood flow and oxygen supply to the heart is vital to improved heart health.

And that is precisely what IF does.

Now, the thing to understand here is that atherosclerosis is not caused by a buildup of plaque and cholesterol in the arteries. They are simply the result of the actual cause, which is damage to the inner layer of blood vessels. And the thing that causes damage is chronic stress.

Chronic stress results not from individual crises in our lives but from a lifestyle that is typified by unhealthy habits. These may include overworking, under sleeping, eating a high carb diet, being inactive all day long, and trying to stay awake with energy drinks and coffee.

Such a lifestyle has many negative consequences on our health but one of the least appreciated is that it damages the endothelium of our blood vessels.

The lack of movement typical of a sedentary lifestyle results in a lack of nitric oxide, which is enhanced through exercise. A key function of nitric oxygen is that it opens up the blood vessels to allow more blood to get into the muscle. It is responsible for the pump effect that bodybuilders experience when blood and oxygen supply to the working muscle is optimized. Diminished levels of nitric oxide contribute to ischemic damage to the arteries. When a lack of exercise is compounded by poor nutritional choices, there are serious impacts upon the blood flow to the heart.

The arterial damage that results from all of this produces an increased release of cholesterol from the liver to help repair the tissue damage in the endothelium. White blood cells also flood into the damaged region to promote healing. These natural healing processes do an effective job of rebuilding the inner lining of the arterial wall. However, this makes the wall thicker resulting in a reduced diameter of open space or the blood to travel through. That means that less blood, and therefore less oxygen, gets to the heart.

You are probably aware that there is a huge focus on reducing cholesterol intake to improve heart health. Doctors prescribe cholesterol-lowering drugs to achieve this. Yet, as we've seen, cholesterol is not the cause of ischemic heart problems. The extra cholesterol is needed to repair the damage that is caused by the real problem.

And what is the real problem? – Poor lifestyle choices.

The strange thing about being prescribed cholesterol-lowering drugs to cure atherosclerosis is that it has recently been shown that statins (the drugs prescribed to lower cholesterol) are contributing to atherosclerosis themselves. This study, which was reported in the journal, **Expert Review of Clinical Pharmacology,** found, *"Statins stimulate atherosclerosis and heart failure: pharmacological mechanisms."*

Despite this, what do you think are the most commonly prescribed drugs in the United States? - Those that are promoted to lower cholesterol! Do not be fooled by the myth that taking cholesterol-lowering drugs will improve your heart health. It won't. But making long term changes to your lifestyle will.

Regular exercise and IF are the real keys to optimizing the functioning of your cardiovascular system.

The study previously referred to that focused on the health benefits of Muslim men during the Holy month of Ramadan had some interesting results specific to the markers of heart health. The lipid profiles across the board showed significant improvement. HDL cholesterol levels (that's the good type) increased while the Total Cholesterol/HDL ratio decreased. The men were also given the D-Dimer test, which assesses the likelihood of forming inappropriate blood clots. The results were way down compared to non-fasting men. There were also decreased levels of CRP, which is another key marker for cardiovascular disease, heart attack, and stroke.

Another study, out of the **American Journal of Clinical Nutrition** looked at the effect of intermittent fasting on heart disease risk factors in obese people. Sixteen obese subjects were put on an intermittent fasting regimen for 10 weeks. The results showed a reduction in body fat percentage, blood pressure, and heart rate. The study's conclusion stated that IF is a, *"viable diet option to help obese individuals lose weight and decrease CAD risk."*

Oxidative Stress/Free Radical Damage

The ill-effects of aging have been directly related to oxidative stress. So, what is oxidative stress?

Oxygen-containing molecules that have an uneven number of electrons are known as free radicals. When we have an imbalance between free radicals and antioxidants in the body, then we are in a state of oxidative stress. Their uneven number allows free radicals to easily interact with other molecules, in effect corrupting them. They can cause large chain chemical reactions in the body. These reactions are called oxidation.

Free radicals can have beneficial effects on the body. They can fight off pathogens that result in infection. But they can only do this when their number is balanced out by antioxidants. When they overpower antioxidants, the free radicals will begin stomping around like a bull in a China shop. Free radicals can damage fatty tissue, DNA and proteins in your body. This damage can result in the following conditions:

- Diabetes
- Atherosclerosis
- High blood pressure
- Heart disease
- Parkinson's
- Alzheimer's
- Cancer

Oxidative stress is also, as mentioned at the outset, a contributing factor to the aging process.
We all naturally produce a certain number of free radicals. The very act of exercising produces them. But other factors which can lead to excess, resulting in oxidative stress, include:

- Pesticides and cleaners
- Cigarette smoke
- Radiation
- Pollution
- A high sugar diet
- Alcohol

Intermittent fasting has a powerful impact on oxidative stress. The main reason is that it leads to the body burning fat rather than glucose as its energy source. Fat burning is a much cleaner form of energy than glucose.

The reason? – Fat burning does not produce as many free radicals as glucose burning does. It's a collateral effect of producing free radicals that is the primary reason that glucose is known as a *dirty* fuel source for the body.

As we've seen, free radicals only become problematic when they out-balance antioxidants in the body. So, increasing antioxidants is another way to prevent oxidative stress. Eating a diet that is rich in raw, organic vegetables and fruits will help to increase your antioxidant levels. Combining this with intermittent fasting will allow for far greater absorption of these oxidative stress defeating antioxidants.

IF itself has been seen to increase the levels of antioxidants in the body. In one study, test subjects put on an intermittent fasting regimen were shown to have higher levels of the antioxidants Vitamin E and Coenzyme Q10. Intermittent fasting has also been shown to increase the levels of what is known as heat shock proteins. Among these proteins are HSP-70 in liver cells and protein-78 in the brain. These proteins help to protect the body against free radical damage.

However, IF's beneficial effects on oxidative stress go further. A report in the journal, *Mechanisms of Ageing and Development*, showed that four months of intermittent fasting significantly reduced oxidative stress and free radical damage. According to the study, the main way it did this was by preventing free radical damage in the first place due to the cleaner energy system that intermittent fasting brings about.

IF also increases the activity of the mitochondria. We can think of mitochondria as the digestive system of the cell. They ensure that the cell is full of energy. When the levels of free radicals are reduced, the mitochondria can do its work far more efficiently. This increases energy levels and leads to increased fat burn.

In this section, we have only scratched the surface of the research showing how beneficial an IF lifestyle is to the health and well-being of the human body. Intermittent fasting has a remarkable curative ability. It will provide the means to cleanse and clear out your system, in the process removing the causes of a whole host of diseases from possibly developing in the body. And, unlike the medications which physicians typically dole out, it does all of this without posing harmful side effects. Furthermore, it is the most effective long-term route to lower body-fat levels.

As a word of warning, if you have any underlying medical conditions or other health concerns you should always consult with your medical practitioner to discuss your IF plans before beginning.

Chapter 4 – The Advantages of Intermittent Fasting Over Dieting

Why You Should NEVER Diet

The conventional wisdom about losing weight hasn't changed for more than a hundred years. That thinking tells us that it is all about calories. If you consume calories above those burned through metabolism and activity, you'll get fat. So, understandably, it makes total sense to believe that to lose that fat, you've got to eat fewer calories and exercise more.

The only problem is that millions of people have been doing just that – and getting fatter! There is a mountain of evidence, both anecdotal and research-based, showing that this approach needs to go on the scrap heap. In this section, we'll take a look at some studies on calorie-reduced diets and why they are not working. We'll then delve into the details of why you must NEVER go on a diet again – ever!

A 2009 study, published in the journal *Lancet*, put participants with an average age of 36 and an average Body Mass Index (BMI) of 35 on a calorie-reduced diet (1,000kcal/4184kJ reduction) for a full 12 months. Half of them also exercised. After twelve months, the results were as follows:

- Diet only group: 0.9kg/1.98lbs lost

- Diet and exercise: 2.2kg/4.85lbs lost

Another 12 months study involved people with an average age of 42 who had an average BMI of 36.5. They were on a diet of between 1,200kcal/5020.8kJ and 1,500kcal/6276kJ per day. Half of them also did regular aerobic exercise and resistance exercise. Here are the results:

- Diet only group: 4.6kg/10.14lbs lost
- Diet and exercise: 5.2kg/11.46lbs lost

A third study had people with an average age of 45, and an average BMI of 36.0 put on a low-fat diet containing 800-1,000kcal/3347- 4184kJ per day. Again, half of them were given exercise in the form of brisk walking for 3 miles, five times per week. This diet lasted for two years. Here are their results:

- Diet only group: 2.1kg/4.62lbs lost
- Diet and exercise: 2.5kg/5.51lbs lost

Our final study involved men with an average age of 43 and an average BMI of 25.5. They followed a low-fat, high carb diet for 12 months. Once more, some of the group added exercise, this time in the form of 30 minutes of aerobic exercise, 4-5 times per week. Results were:

- Diet only group: No change in weight
- Diet and exercise: 1.9kg/4.18lbs lost

Let's now take a look at a summary of those results…

Study	Length (months)	Kg weight change (diet)	Kg weight change (overall)

1	12	-0.9/1.98	-2.2/4.85
2	12	-4.6/10.14	-5.2/11.46
3	24	-2.1/4.62	-2.5/5.51
4	12	0.0	-1.9/4.18
Average		-1.9/4.18	-2.95/6.50

So, what do we learn from these diet studies?

After an average of 12 months of hardcore dieting, the average weight loss was just 2kg/4.4lbs. Even with added exercise to the equation, the weight loss only went up to 3kg/6.6lbs. Keep in mind, too, that the people on these studies had an abundance of professional support and guidance. The bottom line is that traditional dieting methods, those based on caloric restriction, are a fast track to failure.

The Problems With Dieting (And How IF Fixes Them)

There are many problems with traditional dieting. One of the biggest is that they focus purely on weight loss. Just think of the TV show, *The Biggest Loser*. It's all about getting the *scale* weight down. But the scale cannot tell us what type of weight loss is happening – fat or muscle.

You need to distinguish between these two factors. Rather than being concerned about getting the *scale weight* down, you should focus only on losing fat. And a tape measure is better for that!

If you begin an exercise regime to lose fat weight, your *scale weight* may end up increasing. This increase in weight may occur because muscle is five times heavier than fat. As you lose some fat and gain more muscle from exercise, your scale weight is bound to go up – and believe it or not, that's a good thing; we have already seen IF promotes BOTH muscle gain and fat loss.

Another problem with traditional diets is that it is virtually impossible to maintain over the long term. One study followed sixty obese women for 12 months on a restricted-calorie weight loss diet. Although they did lose weight initially (in the range of 9-17lbs/4-8kg in the first eight weeks), none of the women managed to keep it off, and 21 of them ended up heavier than when they started the diet. After two years, 83 percent of the women ended up gaining more weight than they had lost during the diet period.

So, why do most people end up fatter after a diet than when they started. It all comes down to what the scientific community calls the starvation response. The caloric restriction kicks your body into survival mode. It slows down the metabolism and hoards calories much the same way a bear prepares for the lean times of winter. Your body will cling on to fat to see you through the perceived period of starvation. Then when you go off the diet, the slower metabolism and changed hormonal activity that allowed you to *get through* the starvation period will take some time to readjust to the increased caloric consumption, and you will pile on even more body fat.

However, when you adopt an intermittent fasting lifestyle, the body adapts to your fasting pattern with positive hormonal changes. The metabolism does not slow down, and, rather than being hoarded, fat calories become the primary source for energy burn. Besides, the IF lifestyle is not a diet – it is a lifestyle pattern designed for use every day of your life. That means that you never go *off* it, as you would a traditional diet.

Another major problem with traditional dieting has to do with the psychological effects of the practice. When you restrict certain foods, your brain reacts differently to tasty looking food. Studies show that people on a diet are far more attuned to food. They notice it walking through the mall, picking up flavors, and activating their taste bud juices when they see a type of food that they love. This ramps up the temptation factor.

At the same time, the prefrontal cortex, which is the part of the brain that resists temptation, diminishes when you are on a diet.

So, what this means is that while you are trying to avoid unhealthy foods, your desire is increased, and your brain becomes more attuned to seek them out. As a result, your resolve and ability to resist the temptation fly out the window. That creates the perfect storm for a diet disaster!

Contrast all of this with what happens when you undertake the IF lifestyle. Rather than focusing on cutting back on the foods you love, you make a straightforward adjustment and alter the time of day that you consume them. Of course, changing the type of food intake during your eating window to healthier and less fatty/sugary foods is an important factor; it is not the sole focus. Therefore the psychological impact of seeking out foods you can't have is severely negated.

In this section, we have identified three of the significant problems associated with traditional dieting methods. We have also seen how IF overcomes each of those issues. Put this on top of the myriad of benefits to your body that I detailed in the previous section; it is a wonder that people are still following the archaic, proven to fail diets that are still multiplying and infiltrating in the weight loss industry.

And the reason why people still follow diets more than just doing IF?

Well, if you think about it, IF is hard to monetize and, therefore, harder to market into a sexy new fad within the *multi-billion-dollar* weight loss industry. IF is more difficult to monetize because it requires no meal plans, no calorie-controlled food deliveries, no gadgets, and no sexy celebrity-endorsed exercise routines.

All it requires is just a change to the timing of when you eat.

You, however, are now armed with the knowledge that will prevent you from ever falling into the diet trap again. It doesn't matter how many new fad diets are dressed up or how many powerful celebrity endorsements they can get on Instagram; you know they will never give you the results that you desire. But Intermittent Fasting will.

But is this lifestyle really for you? Let's find out?

Chapter 5 – Is Intermittent Fasting For You?

How Will You *ACTUALLY* Benefit From Adopting IF?

The following types of people will especially benefit from adopting the intermittent fasting lifestyle:

Healthy adults – If you are a healthy adult, as determined by your doctor, then intermittent fasting is one of the best health practices that you can undertake.

Adults with type 2 diabetes – For decades, fasting has been a successful treatment in helping to reverse Type-2 Diabetes. There is a wealth of scientific research to establish its integrity in this regard. However, I still strongly recommend consulting with your doctor before adopting the intermittent fasting lifestyle.

High-level athletes – Fasting can be hugely beneficial for high-level athletes. It will speed up post-workout recovery and enhance nutrient uptake. As a result, athletes will build muscle and strength more efficiently.

Vegetarians – Intermittent fasting is ideally suited for people who follow a vegan or vegetarian lifestyle.

Those aiming to be in ketosis – Intermittent fasting dovetails ideally with eating ketogenic (more on that in later).

Being Cautious About Intermittent Fasting

Children – I do not recommend that children under the age of 18 adopt the intermittent fasting lifestyle. However, children who are overweight or obese do need to make changes to how they eat. Help them to cut out sugars and bad carbs and make smarter eating choices.

Immunosuppressed people – Immunosuppressed people may have such conditions as HIV/AIDS, lupus, cancer, etc. Intermittent fasting can benefit them, but they MUST consult with their doctor first.

Pregnant women – There have been no studies that have shown any adverse effects of intermittent fasting on pregnant women. However, as a matter of caution, pregnant women should consult their doctor before beginning with intermittent fasting.

People with eating disorders – Intermittent fasting will help people with eating disorders to become physically healthier. But it will not address the underlying psychological issues that are at the root of their eating disorder. To treat suspected eating disorders, consult with a doctor for further advice.

6 Questions To Ask Yourself Today

1 - How do I deal with hunger?

Fasting will involve daily periods, usually in the last hour before your feeding window, when you will feel hungry. So, ask yourself how you react to hunger. If you immediately succumb to the urge and grab food, then you are going to have to make some serious changes. To be successful at this, you have got to control your hunger, rather than letting it control you. In Part 3, we show you exactly how you can do this.

2 - Am I Patient?

Real, sustained fat loss does not happen overnight. It takes time. Over the first few months, you will have to be patient as you adopt the IF lifestyle. There will be bumps, and inevitably you will eat outside your feeding window, which, of course, will slow down progress. Beating yourself up over this and giving up will not help. So, are you prepared to keep the faith over the first few months and pick yourself up from blips in eating routines, knowing that you are embedding lifelong habits that are for your good?

3 - Have You Got True Grit?

You need to be determined, focused, and gutsy to make IF work. The change to an IF lifestyle is not going to be a cakewalk. At times you will smell and see others enjoying mouthwatering foods, while you know you've still got another 15 or so hours before you can eat again. That can be tough and bring on real hunger pangs. Expect for it to be mentally demanding and be determined to conquer that challenge with true grit.

4 - Are You Also Prepared To Clean Up What You Eat?

There's a saying that you can't out-train a bad diet. It is just as accurate if you modify the saying to you cannot out-fast a bad diet. Before you get started on IF, you should limit or try to cut out the obvious problem foods. These include . . .

- Sugar-laden foods like sweets, chocolates, desserts, and full-sugar soda's/soft drinks.
- Refined (usually white versions) high carb or fried foods like crisps, fries, bread, pasta, and grains.
- Anything labeled a *low fat* alternative.

In the next section, I will lay out specific suggestions as to what foods to eat during your feeding windows to enhance your fat loss and or muscle growth.

5 - Are You Prepared to Exercise?

IF will work for you in the absence of exercise, but you will get so much more out of intermittent fasting if you exercise. That doesn't mean that you have to be running for an hour every day. But you should plan to incorporate a 30minute resistance training/cardio workout into your routine at a minimum of 3 times per week.

6 - Have You Got a Support Network?

To achieve long term success on the IF lifestyle, you will need to have a support network around you. You especially want to have those who share the same living space as you on board. The last thing you want is to have people pressuring you to share a dessert with them when you are two hours into your 18-hour fast.

An ideal scenario would be for your partner or another person in the house to be doing IF alongside you. That way, you can feed off each other's competitive energies and encourage one another to keep going when it gets tough. If family members do not wish to do IF along with you, you should explain it to them, along with all the benefits. Many people think that fasting is a crazy thing to do, so sharing the truth about what it can achieve may well get them on side with what you're doing.

Part Two – Choosing an IF Plan That Works

Chapter 6 – Realistic Intermittent Fasting Methods

In this section, we will examine the different variants of practice that make up IF. The best type of intermittent fasting pattern is the one that suits your lifestyle. So, after having read through them, you may wish to try a few of them out to determine which one works the best for your lifestyle. Choose one plan and give it at least a month's test drive. After that period, if you feel it is not working for you, try another. Remember, these are not diets; they are methods of ratios for timing your eating.

24 Hour Fasts (Eat-Stop-Eat)

The 24-hour fast, more commonly known as eat-stop-eat, involves fasting for a full 24-hour period twice a week. On the remaining five days, you eat as usual, and if you can, a little more responsibly. You do not have to count calories or restrict the number of meals that you eat during the remaining five days.

On this version of intermittent fasting, you do eat something every day. For instance, if you were to fast from 8 am one day until 8 am the next day, then you would eat before 8 am on the first day.

16:8 (Lean Gains)

16:8 or Lean gains is one of the most popular variations of IF. It involves dividing every 24 hours into a 16-hour fast and an 8-hour feeding window. This process allows your body the time it needs to process the nutrients you digest during your feeding window. At the same time, it promotes a fat-burning system for the use of energy by the body.

On the 16:8 Lean gains fasting method, you have the freedom to select the timing of your feeding window. A large portion of that the fasting time will be during the hours that you are sleeping, with many people beginning it after their evening meal at around 7 pm. Starting at this time would take them through until 11 am the following day. Doesn't sound that hard at all, right?

20:4
The 20:4 IF protocol is essentially an extension of 16:8 that pushes the fasted period out to 20-hours, leaving you with just a four-hour feeding window. Many people who follow 20:4, also eat ketogenic during their four-hour feeding window. Users have the freedom to time their fasting and feeding windows to suit their lifestyle.

There is considerable research to show that an extended fasting period will maximize the production of human growth hormone while also encouraging higher fat burn.

Warrior Diet
The Warrior Diet is a modified form of fasting where you do not completely abstain from food throughout the day. You eat a small amount of food for the bulk of the day, and then, in the evening, you can eat an unlimited number of calories.

While not strictly fasting, the warrior diet claims to be based on our ancestral cyclical eating pattern of eating sparingly throughout the day (when hunting most likely occurred) and then eating a lot at night (after they bought home the kill).

The Warrior Diet works from the premise that we should be wholly within the sympathetic system during the day and in the parasympathetic system at night.

The two divisions of the nervous system that are directly affected by fasting are the sympathetic and the parasympathetic nervous systems. The sympathetic system controls the body's fight or flight response to stress. The parasympathetic system regulates the rest and digestive functions of the body. Fasting by eating very little during the day helps to achieve this.

During the *undereating* phase, which takes up most the day, when you are active, very little energy is devoted to the digestive process, allowing more power to be dedicated to detoxifying, cleansing, burning body fat and regulating hormone levels. While in the undereating phase, the only things you eat are raw, fresh produce, and a little protein.

When you pass into the overeating phase, you purposefully eat more than you usually would. But you only do this with your main evening meal. Be sure to get a full complement of proteins, fats, and carbs and eat until you are entirely satiated. You should, of course, be eating healthy foods.

When you overeat after a fast, the body uses those excess calories far more effectively. Studies have shown that the fasted body will:

- Burn fat cells
- Assimilate nutrients
- Build lean muscle mass

- Secrete growth hormone faster when you overeat post fasting

OMAD

OMAD stands for *one meal a day*. It is also known as the 23:1 Method. It involves fasting for 23 hours each day and eating for one hour. Outside of that single hour, you do not eat any food or consume any beverages that contain calories. Within your one-hour eating window, there are no restrictions on what you eat. Of course, it will be far better for a person's overall health to eat healthily during this time.

5:2

The 5:2 Method is known as a modified fasting program. It involves eating, *generally*, for five days of your choosing throughout the week and then restricting your caloric intake to just 500kcals/2092kJ per day for women and 600kcals/ 2510kJ per day for men on the other two chosen days.

The two days of restricted eating do not have to be consecutive. The evening before the first limited calorie day, you should finish eating at 8 pm. The following morning you will have a light snack for breakfast (average 300kcals/1255.2kJ) and then eat nothing throughout the day and then have a similar small 300 calorie snack that evening. The foods that you eat should be low on the glycemic index (low GI foods) to not to spike your insulin level.

With the 5:2 fast, you never go a full day without eating. You also have the flexibility to select which days of the week you fast. However, because you are not going totally food free, you will still get an increase in blood sugar levels. As a result, you will not lose fat as quickly as if you were to go on a full fast.

Some people also find that eating a small meal of five or six hundred kcals actually will make them feel hungrier than if they hadn't eaten at all. Yet, this method can be an excellent way to introduce yourself to fasting before trying a slightly longer method like the 16:8.

36hr Fast

A 36 hour fast involves not eating for one whole day. As an example, you begin the fast after your dinner meal at 7 pm on Day One. You then go through the entire next day with no food. After sleeping on an empty stomach, you begin eating again at 7 am on Day Two. After completing this pattern of eating, it will give you a 36-hour period of fasting.

Longer fasts, such as this one, will speed up all of the benefits that come from fasting that we discussed in the previous chapter. However, they will also increase the risks. Longer fasts may make some people feel sick, nauseous, or head-achy, not to mention the feelings of hunger pangs. They can also, therefore, be a lot harder, mentally, to tackle as well.

42hr Fast

The 42 hour fast is a progression fast for people who have begun with the 16:8 fast, moved on to the 36-hour fast, and then want to extend the benefits even further.

On the 16:8 fast, many people replace their regular breakfast with a glass of water and maybe a cup of black coffee (no milk or sugar). With a 42 hour diet, you stop eating in the early evening of Day One (let's say at 6 pm). You then fast through all of the next day and the night to 6 am on Day Three. At this stage, you have been fasting for 36 hours. However, rather than breaking the fast, you replace it with a glass of water or black coffee and then continue to fast for another six hours. You have your first meal at noon on Day Three to complete 42 hours of straight fasting.

<u>Fast Mimicking Diet</u>
I use the word diet here and in the other fasting methods as it involves not only timing when you eat but also what and how much food you put into your body.

The fast mimicking diet is a modified form of intermittent fasting that allows you to eat small amounts of food rather than completely abstaining as you would on an IF method. The mimic lasts for five days every month. During the five days, you consume 40 percent of your regular caloric intake. Claims have purported that the traditional form of intermittent fasting can be harmful because it does not provide you with a steady flow of electrolytes and nutrients.

Mimicking fasting is designed to trick your body into thinking that it is going on a fast to reap the benefits of fasting without totally restricting your caloric intake. There are several commercial fasting-mimicking diet products available that provide you with full-5 days worth of food products. Here is an example of a day's worth of fasting-mimicking foods:

- <u>Breakfast:</u> Tea and a nut butter
- <u>Lunch:</u> Small serving of vegetable soup and a few kale crackers
- <u>Snack:</u> A handful of olives
- <u>Dinner:</u> Small bowl of soup

<u>Protein Sparing Modified Fast</u>

A protein-sparing modified fast (PSMF) is a very low-calorie fasting diet that is designed to ensure that a person does not lose muscle mass while shedding body fat. There are two phases to the fast.

The first is an intensive phase lasting 4-6 months in which calories are severely limited.

The second phase is a refeeding period. During this phase, calories will gradually increase back to the pre-fast level. This phase lasts for 6-8 weeks.

During the intensive phase, calories reduce to around 800kcals/3347.2kJ per day. Focus is on lean protein food sources such as chicken breast, egg whites, and fish. The aim is 1.2-1.5 grams/0.042-0.-53oz of protein per kg of bodyweight. The fasting method also allows for between 20-50 grams/0.7-1.7oz of carbohydrates per day. The only fat consumed is that which comes naturally with the proteins consumed.

During the refeeding phase, fat and carb calories are gradually brought back while
at the same time reducing proteins.

The protein-sparing fast is a precise fasting method and will not suit many people other than those looking for a particular result of showing off more muscle.

Fat Fasting
The Fat Fast Diet is a short-term intervention designed to help people who are not losing weight to overcome a plateau, most typically those already following a ketogenic diet. It involves dramatically increasing fat intake for three to five days.

It is commonly used by people who have been following a low carb or keto diet, have had a cheat day, and who want to get their body back into a state of ketosis. People who use fat fasting also claim it's useful for losing a few pounds quickly, without hunger or cravings.

The Fat Fast diet involves eating around 1000kcals/4184kJ per day. That is around half the daily caloric recommendations of the American Dietetic Association. 900kcals/3765.6kJ of those come from fat, with the other 100kcals/418.4kJ coming from carbs and protein. The calories are broken up between 4-5 mini-meals over the day.

Be aware if trying this diet that scientific research is lacking, and many believe the weight loss could be just water weight, which will return when going back to a regular diet.

Dry Fasting

Dry fasting is a type of fast that does not permit the drinking of water during the fasting period. Dry fasting is an advanced method that should only be practiced by people who are experienced fasters. However, this does not mean it is a dangerous method either. Millions of people around the world partake in dry fasting every year during Ramadan and other religious observances without consequence.

Dry fasting can be done on any version of a fasting method but is believed to work best with those also following a keto diet. It is easier for those on a keto diet because the body will be able to sustain itself better, and you will not incur as many cravings for food or water. Many believe that dry fasting will accentuate the benefits of regular fasting, but specifically, it is associated with significantly reduced inflammation, lower blood pressure, and balanced glucose.

Juice Fasting

Juice Fasting, also known as Juice Cleansing, involves consuming nothing but fruit and vegetable juices (not like smoothies that have all the *bits*), with no calories in the form of solid food being taken into the body. Juice fasting is widely used for detoxification purposes.

The Juice Fast involves consuming fruit juices and broth. These meals are spread evenly over the day. A couple of sample juice recipes follow:

Pineapple and Pear (Serves 1)

One pear, cored and quartered
One apple, cored and quartered
One slice of pineapple, peeled, including the core
Put all ingredients through an electric juicer, then serve

Veggie Apple (Serves 1)

½ small cucumber
Four carrots, unpeeled
Two celery sticks
One apple, cored and quartered
Put all ingredients through an electric juicer, then serve

The Juice Fast lasts typically for five days. And with only liquid calories consumed, the amount of calories is significantly reduced. You can, however, stop any time short of that if you wish.

Often, Juice Fasts take place over a weekend, when people have more time to prepare and enjoy them. In a study published by Scientific Reports, researchers found that juice fasting increased the amounts of some health-promoting bacteria and lowered the number of bacteria that cause illness.

However, you should be aware that many of the other benefits purported by users of Juice Cleanses are anecdotal, meaning they lack the scientific proof to support them.

Chapter 7 – What To Eat During Your Feeding Windows

Fasting & Eating

The physiological benefits of the fasting process are quite remarkable. During the hours that you are abstaining from food, there are extraordinary things taking place inside your body. However, what happens to you during your eating period is just as important.

I stated earlier that you could not out-fast a lousy diet. The benefits of fasting are so prevalent that you will benefit to some degree from fasting even if you pile junk into your body during your feeding windows. But they will be exponentially better if you eat healthily during both fasting and non-fasting periods.

In this section, we'll break down the confusing and conflicting subject of what you should be eating during your feeding windows.

Habit Based Nutrition

Losing body fat and keeping it off will only happen if you develop sound nutritional practices. These habits need to become as familiar to you as brushing your teeth. Only then will you indeed be able to master your dietary intake. In

this section, I will distill the confusing and often
overwhelming subject of nutrition down into just six habits.

Here's how the six habits will help to put your healthy
nutritional habits on autopilot . . .

- They help guide food selection
- Portion sizes
- No need to count calories
- Timing

By not requiring calorie-counting, the strategy presents a
simple-to-understand and easy-to-apply method of
guaranteeing a well-balanced diet specifically targeted to
active individuals.

The strategy can help establish rules for each meal, thus
directing meal-by-meal nutritional choices and intake.

- **Habit One**

Follow the 1-2-3 rule. In each of your meals, approximately
1 part of the calories should come from fats, two parts from
protein, and three parts from carbohydrates.

Here's an example. Let's say you eat a meal that totals
600kcals/2510.4kJ. If you're following the 1-2-3 rule, each
meal is as follows:

- 100kcals/418.4kJ from fat
- 200kcals/836.8kJ from protein
- 300kcals/1255.2kJ from carbs

- **Habit Two**

The 1-2-3 macronutrient approach is a general guideline.
We can get more specific by thinking about what we will
be doing for the 3 hours after each meal.

We should adjust our carbohydrate intake accordingly. If you are going to exercise, you will want to increase your carb intake. If the next three hours is going to be mostly sedentary, cut back on your carb content.

The following will help you to plan your intake at each meal (the calorie changes should come from carbs).

The meal 3 hours before a:

- <u>Strenuous Workout</u> (requiring all your energy and effort at high intensity for at least 30mins)
  + 300kcals/1255.2kJ to an average meal

- <u>Moderate Workout</u> (50-60% higher heart rate than resting for at least 30mins)
  + 200kcals/836.8kJ to an average meal

- <u>Vigorous Activity</u> (Hiking, carrying heavy loads, jogging, cycling fast)
  + 100kcals/418.4kJ to an average meal

- <u>Moderate Activity</u> (Brisk walking, cleaning, mowing lawn)
  + nothing to an average meal

- <u>Light Activity</u> (strolling, light standing, sitting at a computer)
  - 100kcals/418.4kJ from an average meal

- <u>Relaxing</u> (reading, watching TV, meditating, listening to music)
  - 200kcals/836.8kJ from an average meal

- <u>Total Inactivity</u> (sleeping)
  - 300kcals/836.8kJ from an average meal

Remember, when you overeat at a meal, the excess calories get stored as fat. So, if you skip a meal, do not eat to make up for it, feed only for the type of activity level you are going to be doing.

- **Habit Three**

Eat lean protein with every meal.

Contrary to what you may have heard, additional protein is not harmful or unnecessary. Scientific evidence has made it abundantly clear that a high protein diet is entirely safe. It also appears to be necessary for the best health, the best body, and the best performance. You cannot achieve all three of these results unless you are getting in a healthy dose of proteins.

A complete lean protein is one that contains all of the essential amino acids that the human body cannot produce by itself.

A portion size of protein is visually about the size of the palm of your hand, between 20-30g/0.7-1.05oz. Women should get one portion of protein per meal (20-30g/0.7-1.05oz), and men should get two portions per meal (40-60g/1.4-2.1oz).

Getting the required amount of protein will . . .

- maximally stimulate metabolism
- improve muscle mass
- reduce body fat
- help you to feel fuller longer

Protein Guide

<u>Type:</u>   - Lean, complete protein sources
<u>Timing:</u>   - Eaten with each feeding opportunity

Amount: - 1 serving for women (size of palm) 2 servings for men (size of two palms)
Examples: - Lean meats (ground beef, chicken, turkey, bison, venison, etc.)
                - Fish (salmon, tuna, cod, roughy)
                - Eggs (egg whites, occasional whole eggs)
                - Low-fat dairy (cottage cheese, yogurt, skim cheese, string cheese, etc.)
                - Vegetarian choices (tofu, tempeh, soy burgers, soy jerky, soy sausage, soy   bacon, seitan, etc.)
                - Milk protein supplements (whey, casein, milk protein blends)

- **Habit Four**

Eat vegetables with every meal.

Remember when your mother used to tell you to eat up your vegetables? Well, science has confirmed that she knew her stuff.

Science has demonstrated that in addition to the vitamins and minerals that are packed into veggies, there are also essential plant chemicals needed for optimal body functioning. Even more impressive is the fact that vegetables (and fruits) provide an alkaline load to the blood. Since both proteins and grains present acid loads to the blood, it's crucial to balance these acids with alkaline-rich vegetables and fruits. This is important because too much acid and not enough alkalinity results in the loss of bone strength and muscle mass.

To make a success of this habit, include at least two servings of fruits and veggies per meal. As an example, One medium-sized fruit, ½ cup raw chopped fruit or vegetables, and 1 cup of fresh, leafy vegetables each equal one serving.

It's important to remember that vegetables, when broken down, are primarily carbs. So if you are trying to reduce your carbs, eat less starchy vegetables, grains, and cereals, instead, up the number of leafy greens.

- **Habit Five**

Eat other types of carbohydrates only after exercise.

In other words, you need to earn the right to eat high carb foods by working out first.
Yes, you can eat pasta, rice, bread, and sugary foods – so long as you do two things:

- Focus more on eating whole grain varieties (low GI).
- Save them until 1-2 hours after exercise.

The bottom line is that no exercise = no carbs – apart from those gained fruits and vegetables.

During exercise, your body will deplete its glycogen stores. Following the workout that glycogen needs replaced. That is when you can get away with eating some high glycemic-index carbohydrates.

- **Habit Six**

Eat healthy fats daily.

About 30% of your diet should come from fat – not much less, not much more. More important than total fat intake is the balance between saturated, monounsaturated, and polyunsaturated fats.

A goal of:

- 1/3 saturated (from meat fat, poultry skin, butter, lard, cream, cheese),
- 1/3 monounsaturated (from virgin olive oil, some nuts, avocados),
- and 1/3 polyunsaturated fat (from some nuts, some vegetable oils, oily fish) are recommended.

By balancing out fat intake in this way, optimization of health, body composition, and performance will occur.

While the quantities mentioned might seem intimidating at first, rather than focusing too much on exact measures, your focus should be on just adding more healthy fats. By introducing these to a diet of fruits and veggies, carbs when earned, and lean proteins, your dietary fat intake should balance right out.

4 Questions To Ask To Keep Your Habits On Track

1: Where is the complete protein?
Are you about to eat at least one serving (20-30g) of complete protein? If not, find some protein. Women get one portion, and men get two.

2: Where are the veggies?
Are you about to eat at least two servings of veggies? Prepare them any way you like, but eat them with every meal or snack. (One serving is about ½-1 cup).

3: Where are the carbs?

If you have fat to lose but haven't just worked out, put
down the pasta, bread, rice, and other starchy carbs in favor
of a double serving of fruits and veggies. If you have just
worked out, a mix of carb sources is okay.

4: Where are your fats coming from?

Today you need some fat from animal foods, from olive oil,
from mixed nuts, avocado, and from seeds or vegetable
oils. Spread them throughout your feeding window, but
make sure to add them in.

Foods That Should Form Your Nutritional Foundation

Protein
Meat Eaters and Some Vegetarians

- Lean red meat (93% lean, top round, sirloin)
- Salmon
- Omega-3 eggs
- Low-fat, plain yogurt (lactose-free if you can find
  it)
- Protein supplements (milk protein isolates, whey
  protein isolates)

Vegetarian/Vegans

- Tofu
- Edamame Beans
- Tempeh
- Lentils & Chickpeas

- Plant-based protein supplements (rice protein isolates, pea protein)

Veggies & Fruits

- Spinach
- Tomatoes
- Cruciferous vegetables (broccoli, cabbage, cauliflower)
- Mixed berries
- Oranges

Other Carbs

- Mixed beans
- Quinoa
- Whole oats

Good Fats

- Mixed nuts
- Avocados
- Extra virgin olive oil
- Fish Oil
- Flax seeds (ground)

Drinks/Other

- Green tea
- Liquid exercise drinks (quickly digested carbohydrate and protein)

Focus on Fiber!

For the last 150 years, grains have become a staple of the diet in the Western world. This type of consumption has come at the expense of fiber, as many people now consume chronically low levels.

An immediate result of the lack of fiber in your diet is constipation. Apart from the discomfort that this brings, it also makes it extremely difficult to eliminate toxins from your body. Fiber is a form of carbohydrate. However, the body cannot digest it.

Fiber comes in two different forms – soluble and insoluble.

Soluble fiber is found in the following foods . . .

- Oats
- Oat bran
- Dried beans
- Dried peas
- Nuts
- Barley flax
- Oranges
- Apples
- Carrots

Insoluble fiber in . . .

- Green beans
- Dark green leafy vegetables
- Fruit skins
- Root vegetable skins
- Whole-wheat products
- Seeds
- Nuts

For optimal gut health, you need both types of fiber. Gut microflora from fiber ferments in the small intestine, and this produces short-chain fatty acids. The short-chain fatty acids aid in digestion, absorption of nutrients, and metabolism.

Fiber is also a great way to keep yourself full. That's because it adds bulk to your diet without adding extra calories. Not only will it help you to feel fuller sooner, but because it takes longer than other foods to move through your system, it will keep you full longer.
This is because when fiber fills up your stomach, it stimulates receptors that send messages to your brain that tell you to stop eating.

Soluble fiber also decreases enterohepatic recycling of bile acids, which can lower serum cholesterol levels. Insoluble fiber will add bulk to stools while also reducing colon cancer risk.

An added benefit of soluble fiber is that, when it absorbs water, it forms a gel in the lower intestine. This slows the absorption of blood sugar. This, in turn, leads to lower insulin levels, which makes you less likely to store body fat.

Here's how you will benefit from adapting your diet to include more fiber:

- Increased satiety
- Lowered blood fat and cholesterol
- Reduced risk of colon cancer
- Proper intestinal motility
- Enhanced gut health

When it comes to fruits and vegetables, the majority of the fiber is found in the skin, membrane, and seeds. That's why you need to be eating fruits with the skin on. To benefit your gut health, rebalancing it in favor of fat-blasting Bacteroidetes, you need to take in more than the daily recommended level of 25g/0.88oz.

If you are a woman, aim for 35g/1.23oz per day. If you are a man, aim for 48g/1.69oz per day.

Be sure to drink plenty of water when you eat fiber. You'll need a minimum of eight glasses each day to keep the fiber moving through your system. Water, of course, also help to keep you full.

How To Get More Fiber Into Your Body

Most of us are hopeless at getting fiber into our systems. Yet, upping our fiber levels is absolutely crucial to sorting out our gut bacteria to aid in speeding up the loss of body fat faster.

The following will help you to make smart and healthy replacements so that you can meet your daily fiber goals.

Replace this . . .	With this . . .
1 medium plan bagel	2 slices whole-grain bread
1 cup cooked white	1 cup cooked brown

rice

1 cup mashed potatoes

10 potato chips

1 cup orange juice
drink

1 cup spinach soufflé

1 cup cooked farina
cereal

½ cup cream-style corn

1-ounce/30g jelly
beans

1 cup of corn flakes

1 large fruit leather

1 hot dog

rice

1 cup cooked black
beans

3 cups low-fat popcorn

1 fresh orange

½ cup cooked artichoke
hearts

1 cup cooked oatmeal/
porridge

½ cup cooked mashed
minted peas

1-ounce/30g almonds

1 cup raisin bran cereal

1 cup fresh raspberries

2 tbsp. chunky peanut
butter

Chapter 8 – Building Muscle While Fasting

<u>**Fasting To Promote Muscle Growth**</u>
If you have been trying to add muscle mass to your frame for any length of time, then you will be familiar with the concept of eating frequently. The muscle magazines, websites, and YouTube *experts* have been pushing the *consume protein every 2-3 hours* to prevent muscle loss and keep yourself in an anabolic state for decades.

The only problem is that it's not true.

Our hunter-gatherer forebears went for long periods between meals, as they were out hunting for the food that they would eat. During those periods, they needed to maintain their energy and strength. But if they had been getting weaker, losing muscle and slowing their metabolism because they hadn't eaten for 3 hours, they wouldn't have had the energy to hunt. If that were the case, the human species would have died out a long time ago!

Science has also debunked the frequent eating to maintain muscle myth. When you fast for short periods, your metabolism increases. That's because it is working overtime to break down stored body fat into energy in the form of ketones. The reality is that lean muscle tissue will only be consumed by the body when two conditions exist:

- You are in a state of starvation
- You have almost zero body fat on your body

For the body to go into a state of starvation, deprivation of food must occur for more than 48 hours. None of the intermittent fasting diets recommended in this book involve going for that length of time without eating. However, even if you did go for longer, your body would rely on its stored body fat for energy
before it started attacking muscle tissue, as long as your body fat level wasn't already sitting below 5 percent.

Follow the dietary recommendations outlined in the previous section during your fasting period, and you will also have a plentiful supply of amino acids coursing through your system. This further ensures that you are in a muscle-building (anabolic), rather than a muscle-wasting (catabolic) state. Amino acids are absorbed into the muscle cells slowly. This has the added benefit of keeping you feeling fuller for longer, warding off any hunger pangs.

So, fasting will not lead to muscle loss. But how can you tweak intermittent fasting to promote muscle gain and fat loss?

If you are attempting to gain muscle mass, then you will no doubt be working out with weights. The key to achieving maximum muscle mass while intermittent fasting is that you should **NOT FAST** on the days that you are working out.

You should never force your body to perform resistance exercise when you are in a fasted state. To complete the work that you are demanding of your muscles in the gym, they require full muscle glycogen stores. To achieve that, you need to be consuming calories.

Training in a fasted state does have its place if you are overweight, and your primary goal is to achieve fat loss.

But, when you are working out to build muscle, it is something that you should never do.

During the periods when you are eating, it is essential to focus on taking whole food sources of protein into your body. Ready-made forms such as protein shakes or protein bars can be useful if you are in a hurry. Still, they will not replace the overall health-giving benefits of a cooked whole food meal.

Let's now consider what a week of intermittent fasting for muscle gain might look like.

We are going to base this example on a person following a 20:4 IF protocol. That means 20 hours per day, you will be in a fasted state, and there will be a four-hour feeding window per day. We are also going to assume that the person works out at the gym three days per week, on Monday, Wednesday, and Friday.

Based on the above, the person's week fasting protocol for the week would be as follows:

- Sunday   Fasted
- Monday   Non-Fasted
- Tuesday   Fasted
- Wednesday   Non-Fasted
- Thursday   Fasted
- Friday   Non-Fasted
- Saturday   Fasted

On fasted days, the person's feeding window would be between 3 pm and 7 pm (this can be adjusted to suit).

Let's take a look at how this would work, starting with the weekend:

Saturday: You worked out yesterday, so ate normally until 7 pm. You wake up, immediately hydrate with water and then abstain from food until 3 pm. At that time, you have your first meal of the day. At around 4:45 pm, you have a snack, and your next meal is consumed between 6:30 pm and 7 pm. You then stop eating.

Sunday: You follow the same pattern as the day before. However, when it comes to 3 pm, you are now entering your non-fasted state in preparation for the next day's workout. You eat your first meal at 3 pm, a snack at around 4:45 pm, and then your dinner meal between 6:45 pm and 7 pm. You also have an evening snack between 8:30 pm and 9 pm.

Monday: This is your first workout day of the week. You will be heading off to the gym at 9:30 am. At 7:30 am you have a meal that is rich in complex carbs to fuel your muscle glycogen stores (oatmeal with a banana is a good choice).

You then head off to your workout at 9:30 am. Within an hour after your workout, you have your next meal, with a focus on lean proteins and fats. This meal will feel very filling, and you probably won't feel like eating for another 3-4 hours. So, between 2:30 pm and 3:30 pm, you should have another meal, following the 3-2-1 guidelines outlined in the previous section.

Eat your dinner meal between 6:30 pm and 7 pm. Then you enter into the next 20-hour fast phase.

Tuesday: You worked out yesterday, so ate normally until 7 pm. You wake up, immediately hydrate with water and then abstain from food until 3 pm. During the day, you can keep hydrating with water, mineral water, and black coffee. At 3 pm, you have your first meal of the day. At around 4:45 pm, you have a snack, and your next meal is consumed between 6:30 pm and 7 pm. You then stop eating.

Wednesday: This is your second workout day of the week. You will be heading off to the gym today at 4.30 pm. When you get up, have a breakfast full of low GI foods (Ezekiel bread toast with nut butter, drizzled with honey, is a tasty option). This will help you to feel fuller longer until your mid-morning snack.

Eat some skin on fruit to get some fiber in around 10 am. At lunchtime, make sure you are following the 1-2-3 eating plan, adding extra carbs to match the intensity of workout you have planned. Make it a meal that is rich in complex carbs to fuel your muscle glycogen stores. Grilled chicken, broccoli, sweet potato and quinoa salad with feta cheese is a perfect option for maximum protein, fats, and complex carbs.

Have nature's power bar – a banana, around 3 pm for extra energy and muscle building power.

You then head off to your workout at 4.30 pm. Eat your dinner meal between 6:30 pm and 7 pm, with a focus on lean proteins and fats as you had a lot of your carb intake at lunch. Then you enter into the next 20-hour fast phase.

Thursday: You worked out yesterday, so ate normally until 7 pm. You wake up, immediately hydrate with water and then abstain from food until 3 pm. At that time, you have your first meal of the day. At around 4:45 pm, you have a snack, and your next meal is consumed between

6:30 pm and 7 pm. You then stop eating. Notice a pattern emerging?

Friday: This is your third and final workout day of the week. Depending on when you decide to time your gym workout, plan the types of meals you will be having around this, similarly to how you have on previous workout days earlier in the week.

Note: You may wish to include a workout supplement on your training days. A pre-workout powder that mixes with water taken 30 minutes before heading the gym can get you primed for your training session. Look for a product that provides 200-300 milligrams of caffeine as a stimulant, 5 grams of creatine, and 3 grams of betaine.

<u>Key Muscle Mass Nutrition Tips</u>

- The majority of your carb consumption on training days should take place during your pre-workout meal (an hour before heading to the gym), during the workout, and post-workout (an hour after training).

- For optimum nitrogen retention and maximum glycogen replenishment, aim for 20-40g/0.7-1.4oz of high-glycemic carbs (white bread, short-grain rice, potatoes) and an equal amount of protein pre and post-workout.

- Your post-workout meal should be the largest of the day. This is when your cell's glycogen stores will be depleted, and your muscle fibers are broken down.

- Expect weight fluctuations. During your fasting days, you will be depleting your glycogen stores. However, on your workout days, you will be consuming a decent amount of carbohydrates to replenish your glycogen stores. As a result of this, it wouldn't be abnormal to see an increase of 5-10lbs/2-5kg when you step onto the scale on a workout day. This just goes to underscore a point made earlier; the scales are not the ideal way to judge your success. Looking at yourself naked in the mirror and taking accurate body measurements are though!

During your fasting periods, do not consume any calories at all! Some intermittent fasting programs do allow you to consume such things as MCT Oil, butter, cream, or branch chain amino acids. There is some pretty compelling evidence, however, that even these low-calorie foods will curtail the benefits of a fast.

Chapter 9 – Fasting For Fat Loss

Strategies To Maximize Fat Loss Immediately

In this section, we present you with six strategies you can follow to maximize your fat loss while undertaking IF with the goal of fat loss. They will make your transition into an IF lifestyle far smoother.

<u>The Pantry Makeover</u>
The key to eliminating harmful foods from your feeding windows is, naturally, to remove them from your home. That requires quite a bit of will-power, but until you do, you will continuously have temptation within reach. So, here's what you need to do . . .

1. Empty your pantry and put everything on your kitchen table. Now sort out the good from the bad. You know what goes on the wrong side, but just so that there is no confusion, the following items are included:
   - Sweets
   - Biscuits
   - Pastries
   - Donuts
   - Cereals
   - Sugar
   - Cake
   - Potato chips

2. Once you have sorted your pantry items into two
    piles, you have got to summon up the internal
    fortitude required to throw EVERYTHING in the
    bad pile into the trash. Don't worry that you're
    wasting money by throwing perfectly good food
    away. Or, tell yourself that you'll have one final
    fling before divorcing yourself from the garbage
    food – just bite the bullet and chuck them all out!

    If putting things in the trash doesn't sit well with
    you, take them to the local food bank or donate
    them to a homeless shelter. This way, you will not
    feel wasteful and will get the added benefit of doing
    a good deed on the way to starting your own more
    positive eating journey.

3. Now you are ready to restock your kitchen. Use the
    twenty foods we listed under the Habit Based
    Nutrition section as your guide. When shopping,
    stay away from those products that are labeled as
    Lite, *Reduced Fat*, or *No-Fat* – they are usually,
    instead, loaded with sugar.

<u>Curb Evening Cravings</u>

Want a sure-fire, super-simple, inexpensive way to put an
end to post-dinner snacking and grazing?

It's easy!!! – Thirty minutes after your meal, go and brush
your teeth, using a mint gel toothpaste.

There is some solid research that shows that mint curbs
food cravings. In a 2007 study conducted out of Wheeling
Jesuit University, participants who inhaled mint scent were
less hungry and ate 1,800 fewer calories per day than a
control group. This has led researchers to believe that the

smell of mint affects the part of the hypothalamus that controls satiety.

The fresh, minty taste of toothpaste will also curb your desire for food.

The idea of brushing your teeth in the evening is such an ingrained routine in most of our lives that it already symbolizes an official full stop on eating for the day. This works on both a physical and psychological level. So, simply bring the time that you brush forward a few hours.

Working in tandem with the effects of mint, it works with your logic, years of routine – and your natural laziness. After all, you don't want to have to brush your teeth a second time by eating something after brushing. Also, brushing will remove any remnants of food from between your teeth. It is believed that having tiny bits of food stuck in your mouth keeps the gastric juices flowing, which may lead to food cravings.

Thirst Is Not Hunger

Water is vital to fat loss. There are two underlying reasons that millions of people are unable to make traction on their fat burning quest . . .

- People don't know when they are thirsty
- They are taking in the wrong type of fluid

The body triggers its sensation for food and water-based on diminished energy levels. These two sensations reach the brain together – and most people interpret them to be a sensation just to eat. The body does not send a separate signal for thirst and another one for food. As a result, we often reach for food when we should be reaching for water.

For nearly a hundred years, medical science has sold us a false-hood: You'll know when you need water when your mouth becomes dry.

As a result, millions of people will only consider having a drink of water when they have a dry mouth. In their ignorance, these people have allowed themselves to get into a dangerous state of dehydration.

The medical community has a host of diseases to explain the physical consequences of this mass state of dehydration . . . When all they needed to do was to tell us to drink more water.

Here's why you should never rely on a dry mouth as an indicator of thirst... When chewing and swallowing, the body produces ample amounts of saliva. As a result, the mouth will be swimming in liquid even as the rest of the body is crying out for water!

The body's response to dehydration is to produce the symptoms of what we have come to regard as diseases . . .

- Dyspeptic pain
- Colitis pain
- Asthma
- Appendicitis pain
- Hiatus Hernia
- Rheumatoid arthritis pain
- Low Back pain
- Neck pain
- Anginal pain
- Migraines

The simple truth is that people who suffer from these maladies may not be sick at all, but merely thirsty.

If we could separate the hunger and thirst, then we would be at an immediate advantage in the battle to control our body fat levels and to take control of our health.

Well, we can – and here's how: Drink a glass of water before you eat.

When you do that, you will satisfy the body's need for hydration, and you will prevent yourself from over-eating.

Dealing With Diet Drinks

We've fooled ourselves into thinking that any sort of liquid is a suitable replacement for water. Nothing could be further from the truth.

Diet drinks have become a popular *healthy* refreshment. They have replaced the sugar found in regular bottled drinks with artificial sweetener – aspartame.

Many people think replacing sugar with aspartame will help them lose weight. Unfortunately, it does the opposite. About 90 minutes after taking it into our body, there is a physiological panic which compels us to eat to deliver on the promise to provide sweetness to the body that came with the aspartame.

Bottom line: drink artificially sweetened drinks – eat more.

That's why fast-food restaurants offer free refills – they know it will make you want another burger!

Carry around a bottle of water with you during the evening. Rather than snacking if you're hungry, especially after dinner, take sips of water regularly to keep yourself full. A lot of the time it's just thirst, not hunger, especially after a dinner that is moderate to high in sodium.

Set the target of drinking 64 ounces, or 2 liters, of water per day. That equates to 8 x 8-oz/230ml glasses or four regular size water bottles. This will ensure that your body is adequately hydrated by the time that evening rolls around.

Another Cure For Night-Time Cravings

A huge factor in determining IF success for fat loss will involve mastering your after-dinner cravings.

Packing some gum is a great way to help you do just that. Chewing gum can fill the need for something sweet while giving your mouth something to do. Many people feel a need to be always chewing on something. Chewing gum will curb that whole behavior, preventing you from consuming senseless calories before bed. It will also keep your mind engaged while leaving a tasty feeling in your mouth.

We've already mentioned how mint can help your fat loss efforts. By selecting mint gum, you will be getting more crave controlling bang for your buck.

As well as preventing cravings, chewing mint gum regularly has been shown to reduce a person's overall daily caloric intake. A 2011 study, which was published in *Appetite Magazine*, showed that people who chewed mint gum for 5 minutes an hour for three hours, reduced their snacking behaviors, appetite and had lower total daily caloric consumption.

As a bonus, chewing sugar-free gum will also help to prevent cavities. That's because chewing gum stimulates saliva production. Saliva is vital in preventing cavities. Make sure that the gum you select is sugar-free. Also, do not swallow the gum – spit it out when you're done.

Limit yourself to a single piece of gum each evening.

There is a caveat to the gum weight loss habit. Even though chewing gum is an effective way to prevent after-dinner cravings, you are better off not chewing gum before your meal. A 2014 study out of the University of Buffalo, published in the journal *Eating Behaviors,* showed that after chewing mint gum, people chose to eat smaller quantities of healthy foods over the choice of eating more unhealthy foods. The researchers concluded that the mint flavor doesn't go well with fruits and vegetables, leading people to make unwise eating choices.

Pairing Fasting With Keto

IF and the Ketogenic Diet is an excellent nutritional combination. They both use very similar energy systems in the body. When combined, they can be extremely effective at burning body fat. Fasting uses ketone bodies in just the same way that the Keto diet does. When fasting, you are getting your body to a point where it has no choice but to create ketones from stored body fat to deliver the energy we need to function. In other words, when you are fasting, you are in a state of ketosis.

When following the ketogenic diet, you are, in effect, mimicking fasting. However, you do so without completely eliminating calories – you simply remove those calories that contain glucose. Fasting will provide additional benefits, as we have already discovered, but when it comes to fat loss, keto and fasting are mostly doing the same thing.

So, how can you combine IF and keto for even more significant benefits? If you start on the Keto diet, give yourself a month to really take ownership of the process and then begin adding in elements of IF. Your body will already have made the switch from a glucose burning to a fat-burning system. So, when you start your fast, your body will more rapidly take fat from your stored body fat to create ketones to fuel your energy requirements. That is because you have begun priming the body to utilize fat. When you suddenly deprive the body of dietary fat, it will start to search for stored fat.

How To Keto

The ketogenic diet is a high fat, moderate protein, low carb diet. It is designed to force the body to switch from using glucose from carbohydrates to using ketones from fat as its primary energy source. It does this by restricting the intake of carbs and increasing the amount of fat consumed.

The word ketogenesis means that we burn fat as our energy supply. When fatty acids are broken down, they become ketones. The body can either use glucose or ketones to produce adenosine triphosphate (ATP), which is the body's energy source. Without ATP, we would not be alive. Everything we do is dependent on it.

When we take carbohydrates into our body, it ends up as glucose. The body uses glucose to burn energy and become ATP. When we consume protein, it is broken down into amino acids. Amino acids build and maintain the body. When we ingest fats, they become ketones. Ketones also can produce ATP. The goal of the ketogenic diet is only to use fats as the body's energy source.

The ketogenic diet mimics the effects of fasting. In a fasted state, the body produces ketones, as a result of the body has to burn stored fat rather than carbohydrates. The original ketogenic diet had a fat to protein and carbs ratio of 4:1.

Although the ratios may vary, a typical macronutrient breakdown on the ketogenic diet is 80 percent fat, 15 percent protein, and 5 percent carbohydrate.

Carb Confusion Clarified

Carbohydrates are the body's default macronutrient for energy production. When ingesting carbs, they are broken down and absorbed through the walls of the intestines and then into the bloodstream. In the liver, they become glucose. The insulin that is released when we eat carbs then transports the glucose to the cells of your body, where it is used as the energy to power every breath, movement, both voluntary and involuntary.

Some of the glucose that we don't use immediately can be stored in the liver for future use in the form of glycogen.

This amounts to about 2400kcals/10041kJ or 600g/21oz worth of carbs. The balance will be saved as body fat.

There are two types of carbohydrates . . .

- Simple
- Complex

Simple carbs contain fewer than three molecules. This makes it easy to digest, which delivers a quick energy hit.

Complex carbs are made up of three or more molecules. They take longer to digest, providing longer-lasting energy. Examples of complex carbs are vegetables, whole grains, and potatoes.

Carbohydrates are in a lot of foods, even those that you might not suspect. Even seemingly healthy choices such as whole grains, fruit, and rice are loaded with them. The carbs in these foods will be converted to glucose, just like those that come from refined sugars. They, too, will be stored as body fat if they are not burned off.

In the absence of carbs, your body has an alternate fuel source. This is stored body fat. It does this by converting fat into ketone bodies.

The beauty of ketones is that they can create energy without the use of insulin. As we've already seen, the insulin fluctuations that arise when we eat carbs are a significant contributor to fat gain. By reducing our daily carbohydrate intake to fewer than 20g/0.7oz of carbs per day, we will be able to stabilize our insulin levels. This will, in turn, result in the dropping of blood glucose levels to the normal range, which is between 60 and 100 mg/dl.

Therefore, reducing your carb intake to 20 grams per day is not only safe, but it is also one of the healthiest things you can do to promote fat loss, glucose stability, and energy enhancement.

What Foods Can I Eat on a Ketosis Diet?

The Keto diet takes most other diet plans and stands them on their head. The common denominator of the majority of diets is limited fat intake. With the keto diet, your goal is to eat more saturated fat.

Traditional diets almost universally encourage increased fruit and vegetable consumption. The keto diet cuts out the majority of vegetables and fruits but does allow for a generous amount of green, starchy vegetables such as lettuce and spinach.

Traditional diets are built around caloric restriction. On the keto diet, this is not necessary.

<u>List of Foods Allowed on the Keto Diet</u>
This is not an exhaustive list of foods allowed on a ketogenic diet for weight loss. It is, however, representative of the types of foods you should be consuming. . .

*Fish	*Butter	*Cauliflower
	*Macadamias	
*Meat	*Mayonnaise	*Green beans
	*Water	
*Poultry	*Coconut Oil	*Whipped cream
	*Tea	

*Bacon	*Macadamia Oil	*Cheese
	*Coffee	
*Sausage	*Asparagus	*Whole milk
*Avocado	*Broccoli	*Cashews

Intermittent Fasting FAQ

How long do you need to fast to receive fat loss benefits?

To receive the benefits of IF, you need to have a fasting period of at least 16 hours. That may sound daunting, but keep in mind, it includes the hours that you are sleeping. So, if your last meal were at 7 pm, a 16 hour fast would take you through to 11 am the following day. You would then have an 8-hour window between 11 am and 7 pm during which you would consume all of your calories for the day.

Will Intermittent Fasting rob me of energy?

No, it will not rob you of energy, even though it is logical to think that it would. After all, we get energy from food. So, you would automatically believe if we don't eat, we'll be dragging the chain all day long. However, as we've already discussed, your body has a lot of stored energy just waiting to be burned up. It's probably sitting around your belly area right now. Intermittent fasting provides the trigger to be able to access it.

When I come off a fast, won't I just binge anyway?

Not according to scientific evidence. Dr. Krista Varady, from the University of Illinois in Chicago, conducted a study that put people on a strict calorie limit every other day. Women were restricted to just 400-500kcal/1673-2092kJ, while men were allowed 500-600kcal/2092-

2510kJ. The calories were all consumed at lunch-time. On an alternate day, they were allowed to eat whatever they wanted. The study participants did not gorge themselves on the alternate day. They ate, on average, 110% of their energy requirements. Their results were similar to what would be obtained on a traditional diet.

IF requires that you follow a sensible, healthy eating pattern during your non-fasting time. Stick to this, and you will have neither the urge nor the need to binge.

Initially, there will be a transition period, where you will get a bit of a shock to your system. After all, you're going from a lifetime of eating whenever you get the urge to only eating within a set window. Pretty quickly, though, your body will adapt. In a 2008 study published in the *American Journal of Clinical Nutrition*, researchers studied the effect of fasting on cognition, activity, sleep, and interstitial glucose concentrations. They found that none of these factors were affected by short term fasting.

What are the top tips for fasting?

1. Drink water
2. Stay busy
3. Drink coffee
4. Ride the waves
5. Don't tell people you are fasting
6. Give yourself one month
7. Follow a nutritious diet during your feeding windows
8. Don't binge
9. Fit fasting into your lifestyle

Is fasting safe for women?
Yes, fasting is equally effective for men and women. For

some strange reason, there is a general belief that the practice of fasting will be detrimental to women. However, there is no research or anecdotal evidence to support such a conclusion.

Part Three – Making Intermittent Fasting Work For You

Chapter 10 – The Fasting Mindset

In Part One of this book, we took a close look at the logical, science-backed reasons why IF is one of the healthiest things that you can do for your body. Then, in Part Two, we focused on the practical application of Intermittent Fasting into your lifestyle.

In Part Three, we apply ourselves to what is, arguably, the most critical aspect of all – behavioral change.

Why is it that the majority of people who try weight loss programs, including IF, fail?

It's not that they don't have the will-power. It may not even be because the program is fundamentally unsound. The real reason that people fail is that the program does not address the root cause of their weight gain. These are the behaviors, thought patterns, and habits that are holding back their success.

In this section, we will provide you with the tools you need to break free from the old habits, limitations, and mindsets that have held you back in the past.

Developing The Intermittent Fasting Mindset

Why do so many people fail to lose weight? Did you know people in the United States spend $4.5 billion each year on attempts to lose weight, yet they are getting bigger and bigger by the day? Why is the country wallowing in an obesity epidemic? There is a flood of information about weight loss at our fingertips! And, the U.S is not alone; many other countries around the world are experiencing problems echoing similar stats.

Could the answer be that the majority of people skip, gloss over, or never even think about the most essential part? – Their mindset for effective weight management.

Unless a person gets their mind primed for success, they will fail to achieve their goals, regardless of what else they do.

(You might want to read that statement again – it's pretty profound).

Achieving A Successful Outlook

There are 3 keys to achieving that prosperous mental outlook. Interestingly, these are the very same reasons that the majority of people fail to achieve their weight loss goals.

They are:

- Self-concept
- Readiness to change
- Environmental management

Self-Concept

We are living in an out of control world. People are so busy nowadays that they hardly have time to think – let alone breathe – before they're off to the next appointment, the next pick up or the next thing on their to-do list. As a result, many people accept what happens to them as inevitable, as something over which they have little control, or as pure chance. They pile on weight, fail to stick to an exercise program or ditch their clean eating plan when the pressure comes on like waves. They are being tossed about in an ocean of ill-discipline, self-indulgence, and mediocrity. The truth is very different – Every person, me and you included, has the power to **take control** of their destiny. You are not controlled by circumstance unless you allow yourself. Taking control is especially important when it comes to the most personal and precious thing we possess – our health. A balanced life, one in which we are giving proper attention to maintaining our physical, emotional, spiritual, and psychological health, is within the grasp of each one of us. All we need is the courage to reach out and grasp hold of it.

Sudden weight gain – or sudden weight loss for that matter – is a sign that our life is out of balance. When that happens, we are giving too much emphasis to one area at the expense of another. Too often, the part that gets the sharp shift is our physical health. And yet, our physical health is at the core of our well-being. We may be doing amazing things in the business world, accumulating lots of wealth and or possessions, and building a legacy for ourselves. But what is it all for if we are making ourselves unhealthy in the process?

The cycle of weight gain has psychological roots. Often those roots are embedded in our negative self-talk. We are talking to ourselves all day long – you're probably doing it as you read these words. On an average day, you have some 60,000 thoughts. Most of those thoughts are repetitive thoughts from the day before. . . And the one before that.

Now for the startling part – for most people, the vast majority of those 60,000 thoughts are negative.

For many of us, those negative thoughts manifest themselves as statements of failure. Statements such as, *"I will always be fat,"* or, *"It'll never work because I love food too much."* Learning to re-program our minds to eliminate negativity is key to taking control of our weight.

Another key factor in the weight gain roller coaster has to do with something that the father of sexual psychology, Sigmund Freud, identified over a hundred years ago. He called it the Pleasure Principle.

Freud identified the search for pleasure as a driving force within humans. Our sense of wellness, joy, and aliveness is directly related to the pleasure that we can derive from our daily experiences. Now, here's the rub for those with weight issues. If you're not finding pleasure in other areas of your life, you'll seek substitute pleasures. These substitutes may provide instant gratification but in the long-term, create negative consequences. People may choose alcohol, drugs, or gambling as their replacement pleasure – but the most common substitute is food.

From the above, it is clear that gaining and keeping control of your weight is about a whole lot more than counting calories and doing laps in the pool. Weight loss management has to be part of a total change that incorporates achieving life balance, psychological health, and a positive self-image. The only real way to develop a lean, shapely, healthy body is to develop a mindset for fat loss.

Spend the time to do that and everything else – the physical aspects like exercising and eating – will be so deeply ingrained in your psyche that you will be programmed for success. A lean, healthy body will soon follow.

- **Self -Reflection**

How's your life balance? Can you effectively juggle your work, family, and personal time? Take this quiz to find out.

Respond to each question with a number between 1 and 5, where 5 is always, and 1 is never.

The Home Front

- Do you feel overwhelmed by the responsibilities of running your home?　　1 2 3 4 5

- Do you find yourself bickering over trivial things out of frustration?　　1 2 3 4 5

- Does your family complain that you don't　　1 2 3

spend enough time with them?   4 5

- Do you feel resentful about your family   1 2 3
  obligations?   4 5

Subtotal =

The Work Place

- Do you feel guilty when your work is   1 2 3
  encroaching on your family time?   4 5

- Do you feel frustrated because you don't   1 2 3
  earn enough money?   4 5

- Do you feel annoyed when you have to bring   1 2 3
  work home to complete?   4 5

- Do you often miss meals or make unwise   1 2 3
  food choices due to your work schedule?   4 5

Subtotal =

Getting Personal

- Do you struggle to find time for yourself   1 2 3
  each day/week?   4 5

- Do you feel that you are giving all the time 1 2 3
  and never getting anything back?   4 5

- Do you find time to exercise/relax and just   1 2 3
  chill out?   4 5

- Do you often feel tired in the mid-afternoon 1 2 3
  and wiped out by 8 pm?   4 5

Subtotal =

TOTAL =

How'd you go? If your total is:
20 or less, then you've got a great balance between work, home, and your personal life.
21-30 means that you're doing pretty well but require some tweaking to get the balance better.
31-40, and you need to take a serious look at your priorities.
41-50 means that you're already in free-fall - turn the page and start reclaiming your life!

<u>Find Your Identity</u>

Do you have an identity? Do you have an inner sense of who you are, what you stand for, and what you will and will not allow yourself to do?

When you do, you become armed with self-knowledge that instills confidence and self-belief. You become like a rock of stability, able to control your life rather than allowing other people to control it for you. This, in turn, builds within you the quality of resilience – the ability to let negative comments, hurtful actions, or disappointing experiences wash over you without getting you down. And when you can do this, you develop the vital quality of self-esteem. Without it, you will never reach your weight management goals.

Self-esteem is all about how you feel about yourself. It answers the question, *"How do I feel about who I am?"*

So, how about it? Underneath it all, do you love or loathe yourself?

Do you take pride in your accomplishments every day? Do you pat yourself on the back and acknowledge your achievements?

Do you see yourself as a good person, a compassionate, caring, empathetic human being who tries to do their best in everything?

Or do you beat yourself up over the things that you haven't been able to achieve?

Do you focus on your physical flaws, convincing yourself that you'll never be able to transform your body?

Do you develop insecurities and excessive concerns about what others feel about you?

Do you consider yourself to be a failure?

Are You Ready For Change?

You will never achieve a thriving, meaningful life change unless you love yourself.

Why not? Because, unless you genuinely see yourself as worthy of change, you will subconsciously make efforts to sabotage your goals. You will inevitably find a way to throw a spanner in the works.

Unless you are genuinely convinced that you are worthy of change, you will not change. That is why you need to analyze your self-esteem right now. Unless you see genuine and lasting self-love, you need to work to build your self-esteem before you ever begin a weight management program.

Vital to your happiness is a feeling of self-worth. The following Self-Esteem test will allow you to get an accurate gauge of just how you view yourself:

The Sorensen Self Esteem Test

Place a tick in the box beside each statement that you find to be the truest. Your score is explained after the test.

	Agree	Disagree
⇒ I generally feel anxious in new social situations where I may not know what's expected of me. I find it difficult to hear criticism about myself.		

	Agree	Disagree
⇒ I fear being made to look like a fool.		

	Agree	Disagree
⇒ I tend to magnify my mistakes and minimize my successes.		

	Agree	Disagree
⇒ I am very critical of myself and others.		

	Agree	Disagree
⇒ I have periods in which I feel devastated and/or depressed.		

	Agree	Disagree
⇒ I am anxious and fearful much of the time.		

	Agree	Disagree
⇒ When someone mistreats me, I think that I must have done		

something to deserve it.

	Agree	Disagree
⇒ I have difficulty knowing who to trust and when to trust.		
⇒ I often feel like I don't know the right thing to do or say.		
⇒ I am very concerned about my appearance.		
⇒ I am easily embarrassed.		
⇒ I think others are very focused on – and critical of – what I say and do.		
⇒ I fear to make a mistake that others might see.		
⇒ I often feel depressed about things I've said and done or things I failed to say or do.		
⇒ I have avoided making changes in my life because I was fearful of making a mistake or failing.		
⇒ I often get defensive and strike back when I perceive I'm being criticized.		
⇒ I have not accomplished what I am capable of due to fear		

	Agree	Disagree
and avoidance.		
⇒ I tend to let fear and anxiety control many of my decisions.		
⇒ I tend to think negatively much of the time.		
⇒ I have found it difficult to perform adequately or without embarrassment when involved in sex.		
⇒ I'm one of the following: The person who reveals too much personal information about myself or the person who seldom reveals personal information.		
⇒ I often get so anxious that I don't know what to say.		
⇒ I often procrastinate.		
⇒ I try to avoid conflict and confrontation.		
⇒ I've been told I'm too sensitive.		
⇒ I felt inferior or inadequate as a child.		
⇒ I tend to think that I have		

	Agree	Disagree
higher standards than others.		
⇒ I often feel like I don't know what is expected of me.		
⇒ I often compare myself to others.		
⇒ I frequently think of negative thoughts about myself and others.		
⇒ I often feel that others mistreat me and/or take advantage of me.		
⇒ At night, I frequently review my day, analyzing what I said and did or what others said and did to me that day.		
⇒ I often make decisions based on what would please others rather than what I want or without even considering what I want.		
⇒ I often think that others don't respect me.		
⇒ I often refrain from sharing my opinions, ideas, and feelings in groups.		
⇒ I sometimes lie when I feel		

	Agree	Disagree
that the truth would result in criticism or rejection.		
⇒ I'm fearful that I will say or do something that will make me look stupid or incompetent.		
⇒ I do not set goals for the future.		
⇒ I am easily discouraged.		
⇒ I am not very aware of my feelings.		
⇒ I grew up in a dysfunctional home.		
⇒ I think life is harder for me than for most other people.		
⇒ I often avoid situations where I think I will be uncomfortable.		
⇒ I tend to be a perfectionist, needing to look perfect and to do things correctly.		
⇒ I feel too embarrassed to eat out alone or to attend movies and other activities by myself.		
⇒ I often find myself angry or		

	Agree	Disagree
hurt by the behavior and words of others.		
⇒ At times I get so anxious or upset that I experience most of the following: heart racing or pounding, sweating, tearfulness, blushing, difficulty in swallowing or lump in my throat, shaking, poor concentration, dizziness, nausea or diarrhea, butterflies.		
⇒ I am very fearful of criticism, disapproval, or rejection.		
⇒ I rely on the opinions of others to make decisions.		

YOUR SCORE
Add up all the agrees you ticked:

- **0 – 4** = You have relatively good self-esteem
- **5 – 10** = You have mild low self-esteem
- **11 – 18** = You have moderately low self-esteem
- **19 – 50** = You have severely low self-esteem

It's important to realize that your score on this questionnaire in no way indicates that you are not a quality person. Instead, what it does is measure how you view yourself.

If you have a healthy view of yourself, your score will be low.

If your view of yourself is unhealthy, your score will be high.

(Test By Marilyn J. Sorensen, Ph.D., Clinical Psychologist, and Author. Adapted from her book, Breaking the Chain of Low Self Esteem.)

Self-Esteem Builders

Your analysis may have identified a need for improvement in your self-image. The following five steps will help you to turn around your lagging self-esteem:

1. **Identify Your Strengths:** Knowing your skills and traits will give your confidence a boost. Write down three skills and three character strengths that you possess (for example being dependable, empathetic, compassionate).

2. **Identify Your Weaknesses:** By identifying the weak link in your chain of self-esteem, you'll know where you need to fortify yourself. What trait would you like to change about yourself? What do you need to keep a handle on? Is it that you allow silly little things to get on top of you? Do you let your inner voice to talk you out of action? Are you prone to construing cynical motives to the efforts of others?

3. **Know Your Center:** Know what you stand for and be always faithful to it. Do your own thing

regardless of how popular it is with the crowd. Never compromise your values and standards to fit in.

4. **Choose Your Associates Wisely:** Negativity is contagious. If you surround yourself with people who lack drive, ambition, and self-love, then that is what you will get from yourself. The people you need around you are those who will appreciate you, encourage and respect you.

5. **Slam on The Brakes:** When you identify yourself slipping into negative territory – condemning yourself, using negative self-talk, wanting to give up – do something about it immediately. Pull yourself up – tell yourself to stop being stupid and get your head back in the game – because you are better than that!

Environmental Management Through Neurolinguistic Programming

When you decide to begin the IF lifestyle, you commit to making quite a radical change in the way you eat to achieve the outcomes that you want. But for it to succeed, you need to do certain things to make your mind over to this new eating pattern.

Before people decide to jump on board with IF, they mull it over. Part of them really wants to do it. They've seen the results in others, and they've processed all of the factual evidence that it does work. But there is another part of them that is a little worried. They have doubts . . .

- Can I really do this?
- Is this lifestyle possible for me?
- Is it going to be too difficult?

The person has a conflict. Before they can make progress, they have to resolve that conflict. If the conflict persists, they will falter, only doing IF for short bursts and then reverting to their old way of eating. That conflict **MUST** be dealt with at the very outset.

So, let's do that now.

Put both open hands out in front of you. Now look at one side and think of all the reasons you want to do Intermittent Fasting. Think of your health and vitality and how healthy, happy, and secure you will be when you lose the excess body fat. Think too of your reasons for wanting to do IF. It may be to look good for your partner or to be healthier to play sport with your kids.

This is the part of you that wants to do this. Look at your hand and thank yourself for wanting to improve (you don't have to do it out loud, it might sound a little weird!).

Now, look at your other hand. These are all the reasons that you want to sabotage your progress. These are the doubts, fears, and negative thoughts. However, this hand simply wants you to be happy, just like the other hand.

Look now at both hands and realize that the part of you that wants to do it can reassure the part of you that has doubts. That you will be even healthier in the long run if you go for it – you'll be more attractive, more dynamic, and more able to do what you really want to do.

As you look at these two parts, you realize that they both want the same thing. When you allow yourself to start doing the things you need to do to be healthier and happier, then you can bring the two sides closer together. This process will take some time, subconsciously, as your mind works out the details. As the two parts come together, your resolve will become unstoppable.

Both sides are stronger when they work together. The part of you that used to sabotage you, now wants you to succeed. And the part of you that wants you to succeed, just wants you to be happy.

Together they form a new you. Never again will you want to get off base. Never again will you want to stray from the path.

You are on your way!

Follow this technique once a day over the first two weeks of your transition to IF. By then, you will have decided in your core that you are an intermittent faster for life.

Unlearning False Behaviors Fast

To make a success of IF, you have to unlearn some malicious behaviors. From our earliest years, we are conditioned to believe that we have to eat three meals per day. We have been raised that breakfast is the most important meal of the day. But, did you know that this piece of wisdom was invented by cereal companies?

So, let's analyze these beliefs.

A couple of thousand years ago, there was no refrigeration, canning, or another way to store food for long periods. So, when you got up in the morning, there was no coffee, toast, bacon, and eggs or hash browns waiting. You may have had some water, and then you would have to go out and forage for your food.

We see from this that our bodies were meant to intermittently fast. It makes your system more efficient. Eating the way that we've been conditioned is counter-productive to the way our bodies intended to work.

When you begin to eat the way that we were designed to eat, you will start to enjoy the feeling of being hungry. That concept seems strange to most people. We have been conditioned to consider hunger as the enemy. As soon as we feel it, we have to overcome it.

But when you start to enjoy feeling hungry, you can ask yourself, *"Am I really hungry?"* or, *"Am I bored or angry or upset?"* Most of us are disassociated from our physical selves so much that we don't even know if we're physically hungry anymore.

If people could be trained only to eat when they are physically hungry, the obesity problem would be solved overnight. We have been brainwashed into having to eat at breakfast, lunch, and dinner times, whether we are hungry or not. And other people will pressure us to do so.

When you IF, you are learning to enjoy the feeling of hunger as you learn how your body works. When you get into the consciousness of real appetite, then you can dismiss the false hunger. No longer will you be soothing emotional needs with food. When you can do that, it will free you in a way that you never thought possible.

Another benefit of learning only to eat when you are physically hungry is that you will eat less. No longer will you be shoveling food into your mouth that your body doesn't need and so will not burn off. Instead, you will be making your body far more efficient.

How To Overcome Cravings

Contrary to what many people think, conquering cravings is not about increasing your will-power. . . It's about improving your **WON'T POWER!**

That means creating a power state that is so formidable that the old behavior doesn't stand a chance.

I'm about to reveal a potent technique used by elite athletes to get and stay in a power state.

<u>Finding Your Power Circle State</u>
Believe me, this REALLY works, but you've got to do it exactly like this . . .

Imagine a circle in front of you on the floor. This is you in your power state. Ask yourself:

- What color is the circle (the first color that pops into your mind)?
- What sounds do you hear (applause? affirmations? your power song?)
- What feelings (control/focus/energy)?

Now take a deep breath and think about a day in your life when you were at your very best.
You nailed whatever you were doing and felt like a winner.

Now see yourself stepping into that circle and breathe it all in. You are absorbing all of that power, control, focus, and drive, and you are becoming totally unstoppable.

Now open your eyes and imagine that you are at a restaurant. There are temptation foods all around you.

Then you step into your power state.

All of that determination, energy, and laser focus wells up inside you.

Now you don't even notice those temptation foods.

They don't apply to you – they are for lesser, weaker beings.

The power circle technique will allow you to crush your cravings. When you go into that state, cheating will never become an option, and you will have eliminated the biggest hurdle to fasting success!

Discover the power for yourself – it'll turn you into an unstoppable IF/Keto cyborg!

Boosting Your Results

To increase your results on an IF/Keto eating plan, you need to be able to eat less and enjoy it more. Here is a neurolinguistic programming technique to allow you to do just that.

Take a deep breath and close your eyes… Now imagine that it is six months from today.

You are at your ideal weight, having achieved the body fat percentage you wanted. You've added the desired amount of lean body mass, and your muscles are defined.

You also have the mental clarity and all the hidden benefits that come with following the intermittent fasting lifestyle.

From your vantage point six months down the line, you look back on today and realize that you had to make some changes to get there.

Now realize how easy it was to make those changes.

You incorporated a ketogenic plan where you lowered your carbs to twenty grams per day, increased your healthy fats, and moderated your protein intake. You also taught yourself to eat less and enjoy it more.

Now run a movie in your mind of yourself going through a day focused on the intermittent fasting/keto lifestyle. You go for twenty hours without eating and then effortlessly follow a very low carb, high fat, moderate protein eating pattern for the next four hours. You marvel at how easy this process is.

As you watch that movie with all of those future benefits, you realize how easy it was – you hear it, feel it, and experience it.

Now run the movie faster – see it, hear it, feel it. Then jump to the future and look back on today – you realize that today is the day that you made the decision. Today is the day that you did what you needed to do to make this path possible. That today, you know you are on your way to that destination. You have created a mental loop where it is impossible to get off that track.

The more you try to go backward, the more you are driven forward.

Go through this mental rehearsal daily to strengthen your conviction and boost your progress.

How to Enjoy Fewer Options in Your Diet

When you follow an IF/Keto lifestyle, you will have fewer options in your diet than if you were to eat whatever you wanted. There are two ways to view this. You could consider it is limiting your choices. OR you could have the mindset that you are opening up your options for better health, physical activity, and all the other things that you want.

Our brains can screen out all the things that are not important to us. At the same time, the mind focuses on the things that we consider to be important.

It often happens when we have decided to buy a new car. Let's say we want a Corvette. Over the next few days, we'll see Corvettes everywhere we look. Yet, the day before you fixed your heart on that type of car, you probably wouldn't have even noticed if your neighbor had pulled up in a gleaming Corvette Stingray. This can happen with anything that we consider to be important to us.

We can use this ability to train our brain so that when we look at the food options that are not part of our new healthy eating plan, we don't see them.

Here's how to do it . . .
Close your eyes and imagine that you are in a restaurant. You open up the menu, and you don't even notice all the things that used to get your attention. They're not vital to you – they're gone! If you don't see them, you won't want them.

Suddenly, your mind focuses on a laser beam on the things you want – the foods that fit into your IF/Keto lifestyle.

All of the foods that don't fit your lifestyle are blurry – you can't read the words, and the images are unclear.

Now open your eyes, blink a couple of times and then close them again. This time, imagine that you're in the mall and you pass by a café. All of those sweet treats that used to tempt you don't even register in your mind. Instead, your attention goes directly to the foods that you know are going to support your goals.

You can also capitalize on the way that your brain is codified to implement another powerful neurolinguistic technique that will cement in your good eating habits.

You have a part of your brain where things are no longer real for you and another section where things are true for you. An example could be that you used to live somewhere, but now you live somewhere else. The things that were formerly true for us are now no longer real. We can use this mechanism to flip our minds into what we want.

We do this by taking the foods we no longer want to eat and put them in the category that is no longer true for you. You then think about the foods you want, and you flip them into the part of your brain where this is true for you now . . . You follow the IF/Keto lifestyle.

Another handy phrase to use within your mind is . . . That doesn't apply to me.

When you see food items that are on your no-go list – the sweets, sodas, and junk food – simply remind yourself that those foods do not apply to you.

Self-Image Self-Assessment

By the time the average young woman graduates from High School, she will have watched over 22,000 hours of television. That's nearly two and a half years of sitting in front of the TV 24/7. And during that time, she will have been deluged with images of sexy women with perfect bodies.

For many young women, this constant exposure to the perceived body ideal leads to a deep-seated subconscious connection; attaining a Sports illustrated Swimsuit body equals love, happiness, and fulfillment.

And all of this has led to a distorted view of body image among many women. In a recent survey, 41% of female respondents described themselves as too fat, and 29% said that they were currently dieting. Only 17% of them were overweight according to body fat caliper testing.

The results of all of this media-fed body image control are that women have morphed their view of how they think they look onto their total self-image. A less than ideal self-body image can result in some pretty toxic ideas about one's worth. Unless you consider yourself as physically acceptable, you're likely to feel powerless, unworthy, and unloved.

That's pretty harsh when the view of what is acceptable is, in itself, an artificially constructed illusion. After all, the images we see in the magazines are airbrushed and photo-shopped to create an illusion of bodily perfection that simply does not exist. That's why most of us are looking at our body images through a distorted mirror.

The following steps will help you to correct your view:

- **Retrain your brain:** Start retraining yourself to forget about the false images that society has embedded in your mind about the body ideal. It has been designed for one thing only – to take your money. Your body is unique to you – focus on improving it bit by bit and forget everything else – and stop comparing yourself to others.

- **Be kinder and respectful:** Judge your body by what it does for you rather than what you think it looks like. Your body is a fantastic living machine that deserves your respect. Cherish it, feed it so that it can do its best, and NEVER put anything into it that will cause it damage.

- **Create more understanding:** Uncover the real reasons behind any ongoing body image hang-ups that you have. What is it that is holding you back from feeling good about yourself? Could it be that you were never praised as a child? Do you expect perfection from yourself? Whatever the issue is, make up your mind here and now to confront it rationally in the cold light of day. Acknowledge it. Accept it. Then remedy it.

- **Adopt a positive power base:** You are about to engage upon an excellent weight management program that will allow you to achieve your physical goals finally. The mindset that you take into this endeavor is critical. Rather than coming from an, "I'm broken and I need to be fixed," perspective, you should adopt the view that "I'm awesome and I deserve to be the best me that I can be."

- **Don't sweat the small stuff:** Learn to judge yourself by what is important. At the end of the day, your character is more important than your belly size. Develop the qualities of love, compassion, empathy, hospitality, and judge yourself against these criteria. So, make a list of positive non-body traits that you appreciate about yourself. Keep this close by and refer to it every day.

- **Realize that you are not alone**: Everybody has doubts about how they look – including those supermodels who you've probably been judging yourself against for so long. Without their million-dollar make-up and airbrushed photo-shoots, they're just like you.

- **View yourself as a whole person**: You're more than just a sagging butt. Look at yourself naked in the mirror and focus on the bits that you do like (come on, there must be something!)

- **Surround yourself with positivity:** Get closer to positive people who love themselves, and will encourage you in the same regard. These people should love you for who you are, not what you have or how you look.

- **Be stronger than your negative thoughts:** Shut them down, boot them out, and clear the space for positivity. Any time you see a negative thought taking root, squash it, and put a positive affirmation in its place.

- **Treat your body:** Take a soothing bubble bath. Have a relaxing nap. Just find some time to chill out. Give back to the body that, up until now, you've probably been berating and taking for granted.

Where Are You Going?

Most people spend more time planning a party than they do planning their lives. Yet, without a plan and, more specifically, an end goal, our lives will be like waves tossed about on a sea of uncertainty. It would be like playing a game of basketball with no hoops – not only would that be frustrating; it would also be pointless.

It is vital, then, that we start our weight maintenance program with the end in mind. That means establishing just what your ultimate goal for your body is. When this is adequately formulated and planted in your subconscious mind, it can provide direction and acceleration to your forward movement as you transform your goal into reality.

Most people are afraid to set big goals. They have convinced themselves that they are not worthy of them, that they only apply to others who have more talent, natural ability, or inner drive. After all, low expectations are all around us. They are a part of the politically correct climate that prevails in our society. We're told not to set our kids up for failure, to expect mediocrity, and to celebrate the mundane.

That type of thinking does not belong in your mental tool-box.

People may tell you that you need to be realistic, that you're too old, too busy, or too unorganized to succeed. If they do, you need to take that negative energy and flip it, use it to serve as fuel to fire your ambition. Don't be one of those people who get scared by goals and, therefore, only set a goal to the level of what they think they can comfortably achieve – not what they want. Those people end up with weak goals. And soft targets will not stir your passion. Far better to take to heart the words of architect Daniel Burnham:

"Make no small plans; they have no magic to stir your blood to action. Make big plans, aim high in work and hope."

Even though it's essential to set realistic goals, I am a firm believer that there are no unrealistic goals, only unrealistic timelines. Imagine if Arnold Schwarzenegger was told that his goals – to become the best bodybuilder, the highest-paid actor, and a political leader – were unrealistic. Or if Barak Obama's aim to be the first Black US President was unrealistic. Greatness is achieved by people who set unrealistic end-goals – and then set a realistic timeline toward their attainment…

- Be that person.
- Set a big end goal.
- Make sure it's one that excites you and even scares you a little.

If you feel like pulling back to safety and constricting your goal – DON'T!

Be the person who steps up to the plate, not the one who sneaks to the back of the line. You deserve to grasp hold of what you want, not to meekly cling to what you think you deserve. So, think about the body that you really, really want – even if it means shedding a hundred or more pounds.

Focus on what that new you will be like.

Create a specific image in your mind of the end-goal you. See yourself slipping into a bikini and confidently hitting the beach. Look down at your rippling abs; run your hand over them; flex your thighs and glutes. More importantly, focus on what that new you will feel like. . .

- The confidence.
- The self-assuredness.
- The feeling of energy, strength, and power that exudes from the new you.
- The sex appeal.

Imagine how much more focused, more disciplined, and more connected, you will feel. Imagine how confident you will feel in your skin once you have achieved your end-game goal.

Your end-game goal answers the question, "Where Are You Going?" It is the basis from which you will set all of your other goals. These are all stepping-stone goals which will lead inevitably to your end-game goal. You need to keep your end-game goal in focus every day. But more than that – you need to live your life as if that end-game goal has already been accomplished.

Believe in its achievement with such certainty that, to you, it has already happened. By doing so, you will be feeding your subconscious with the altered reality. The modified truth being that you are already at your end-goal – and it will respond with habitual behaviors that will propel you there at warp speed. You will also be able to cultivate the positive emotions that will be part of your end-goal achievement right now. You will be carrying yourself taller, maintaining eye contact when you converse, and feeling in control. And you will love yourself.

End-Goal Checklist

√ Set your ultimate goal - be brave, be bold, and don't sell yourself short.
√ Make up your mind that you will do whatever it takes to achieve your ultimate goal.
√ Work backward from your ultimate goal to establish stepping stone goals.
√ Visualize yourself having already attained your ultimate goal.
√ Live your life as if your ultimate goal has already been achieved.

Strategies For Overcoming Obstacles

- Portion Control.
- Use smaller plates and bowls.
- Have a glass of water before you eat.
- Assess your hunger and fullness before you eat.
- Start eating last so that you eat less socially.
- Don't assume that a packet, tin or jar is a serving.
- Separate leftovers into small containers to avoid being tempted to eat everything in one go.
- Eat fruit before you snack.
- Eat the salad first.
- Reduce Sugars & Sweets.
- Tell others about your new healthier eating habits and ask them for help.
- Use a shopping list when shopping.
- Avoid making food choices when hungry.
- Find a menu planning app.
- Create a menu for each week ahead of time.
- Ask yourself if you need that unhealthy option.

- Remind yourself that everything you put into your body will make you better, or it will make you worse – which do you want?

<u>Ending Emotional Eating</u>

- Keep a food journal, recording what you eat and why.
- Develop new habits (walking, playing cards) that keep you busy during the times that you were most likely to eat emotionally.
- Concentrate on what you are eating.
- Remove tempting food from your home.
- Recruit support from others.
- Understand your emotions.
- Ask yourself, "Can it wait?"
- Write a triggers and solutions list.
- Get a good night's sleep.

Become An Intermittent Faster For Life

Throughout the pages of this book, I have presented a strong case for Intermittent Fasting. You have discovered that it is the most scientifically sound, physiologically balanced, and results-producing fat-loss method that exists. You have also found that there is a perfect nutritional plan to complement Intermittent Fasting… the Ketogenic Diet.

When put together, Intermittent Fasting and the Keto Diet can supercharge your fat loss. I've shown you that the IF/ Keto combo will…

- Burn off fatty tissue 24/7.
- Get and keep your body into a state of ketosis.
- Use fat as your preferential energy burning system.
- Improve insulin sensitivity.
- Boost brainpower.
- Decrease oxidative stress.

But more than that – I have also shown you precisely how to incorporate Intermittent Fasting into your busy, modern lifestyle. You have the strategies to make it work, taking the confusion out of nutrition by breaking it down into six key nutritional habits to follow during your feeding windows. You also have everything you need to integrate the keto diet into your Intermittent Fasting lifestyle to fast-track the success of fasting for fat-loss.

This book has also done what very few weight loss books dare to… It has addressed the elephant in the room when it comes to changing eating habits – ingrained and self-sabotaging behaviors. You have been shown how to improve your thoughts and beliefs about what you can really accomplish.

You can stay committed to your healthy lifestyle change by getting rid of self-limiting beliefs that may have previously been holding you back. You have also become empowered with powerful neurolinguistic programming techniques designed to overcome stress, powerful old habits, and other negative factors that can pop up and hold you back from reaching your true potential.

In short, the pages of this book have given you the tools needed to transform your physique, health, and overall well-being.

I'd now like to conclude with what may be the most relevant statistic of them all… **83 percent**!

That's the percentage of people who read weight loss books and then do absolutely nothing with what they have learned. It's not that they don't agree with what they've read. Instead, they simply fail to take their new-found knowledge and transform it into action.

So, the question facing you is this… What are you going to do with the information that has been presented to you in this book?

Are you going to be like the 83 percent who do absolutely NOTHING…?
OR
Are you going actually to apply what you've learned?

Are you going to apply the clear direction I've provided on

nutrition, to take control of your waistline and your taste-buds finally?
OR
Are you going to sink back to the comfortable – but destructive – relationship that you've always had with food?

Are you going to transform your mental landscape, energizing it with the power of neurolinguistic programming and positive thinking to catapult you forward like an unstoppable machine?
OR
Are you going to languish in a world of stinking thinking, convincing yourself that you are unable to lose weight, get in shape and make traction in your life?

The choice is *yours.*

I challenge you to make the right one!